CONSCIOUSNESS AND THE SOCIAL BRAIN

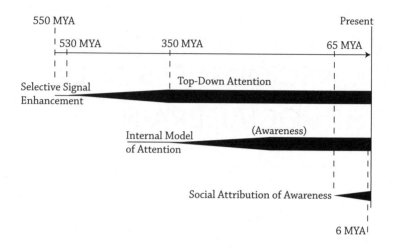

SPECULATIVE EVOLUTIONARY TIMELINE OF CONSCIOUSNESS

The theory at a glance: from selective signal enhancement to consciousness. About half a billion years ago, nervous systems evolved an ability to enhance the most pressing of incoming signals. Gradually, this attentional focus came under top-down control. To effectively predict and deploy its own attentional focus, the brain needed a constantly updated simulation of attention. This model of attention was schematic and lacking in detail. Instead of attributing a complex neuronal machinery to the self, the model attributed to the self an experience of X—the property of being *conscious* of something. Just as the brain could direct attention to external signals or to internal signals, that model of attention could attribute to the self a consciousness of external events or of internal event. As that model increased in sophistication, it came to be used not only to guide one's own attention, but for a variety of other purposes including understanding other beings. Now, in humans, consciousness is a key part of what makes us socially capable. In this theory, consciousness emerged first with a specific function related to the control of attention and continues to evolve and expand its cognitive role. The theory explains why a brain attributes the property of consciousness to itself, and why we humans are so prone to attribute consciousness to the people and objects around us. Timeline: Hydras evolve approximately 550 million years ago (MYA) with no selective signal enhancement; animals that do show selective signal enhancement diverge from each other approximately 530 MYA; animals that show sophisticated top-down control of attention diverge from each other approximately 350 MYA; primates first appear approximately 65 MYA; hominids appear approximately 6 MYA; *Homo sapiens* appear approximately 0.2 MYA

Consciousness and the Social Brain

Michael S. A. Graziano

OXFORD
UNIVERSITY PRESS

OXFORD
UNIVERSITY PRESS

Oxford University Press is a department of the University of Oxford.
It furthers the University's objective of excellence in research, scholarship,
and education by publishing worldwide.

Oxford   New York
Auckland   Cape Town   Dar es Salaam   Hong Kong   Karachi
Kuala Lumpur   Madrid   Melbourne   Mexico City   Nairobi
New Delhi   Shanghai   Taipei   Toronto

With offices in
Argentina   Austria   Brazil   Chile   Czech Republic   France   Greece
Guatemala   Hungary   Italy   Japan   Poland   Portugal   Singapore
South Korea   Switzerland   Thailand   Turkey   Ukraine   Vietnam

Oxford is a registered trademark of Oxford University Press in the
UK and certain other countries.

Published in the United States of America by
Oxford University Press
198 Madison Avenue, New York, NY 10016

Library of Congress Cataloging-in-Publication Data
Graziano, Michael S. A., 1967–
Consciousness and the social brain / Michael S.A. Graziano.
    pages cm
Includes bibliographical references and index.
ISBN 978–0–19–992864–4
1. Consciousness.   2. Brain.   I. Title.
BF311.G692 2013
153—dc23
2012048895

9 8 7 6 5 4 3
Printed in the United States of America
on acid-free paper

For Sabine

Contents

Acknowledgments

Many thanks to the people who patiently read through drafts and provided feedback. Thanks in particular to Sabine Kastner, Joan Bossert, and Bruce Bridgeman. At least some of the inspiration for the book came from Mark Ring, whose unpublished paper outlines the thesis that consciousness must be information or else we would be unable to report it. Some of the material in this book is adapted from a previous article by Graziano and Kastner in 2011.

CONSCIOUSNESS AND THE SOCIAL BRAIN

PART ONE

THE THEORY

1

The Magic Trick

I was in the audience watching a magic show. Per protocol a lady was standing in a tall wooden box, her smiling head sticking out of the top, while the magician stabbed swords through the middle.

A man sitting next to me whispered to his son, "Jimmy, how do you think they do *that*?"

The boy must have been about six or seven. Refusing to be impressed, he hissed back, "It's *obvious*, Dad."

"Really?" his father said. "You figured it out? What's the trick?"

"The magician makes it happen that way," the boy said.

The magician makes it happen. That explanation, as charmingly vacuous as it sounds, could stand as a fair summary of almost every theory, religious or scientific, that has been put forward to explain human consciousness.

What is consciousness? What is the essence of awareness, the spark that makes us *us*? Something lovely apparently buried inside us is aware of ourselves and of our world. Without that awareness, zombie-like, we would presumably have no basis for curiosity, no realization that there is a world about which to be curious, no impetus to seek insight, whether emotional, artistic, religious, or scientific. Consciousness is the window through which we *understand*.

The human brain contains about one hundred billion interacting neurons. Neuroscientists know, at least in general, how that network of neurons can compute information. But how does a brain become *aware* of information? What is sentience itself? In this book I propose a novel scientific theory of what consciousness might be and how a brain might construct it. In this first chapter I briefly sketch the history of ideas on the brain basis of consciousness and how the new proposal might fit into the larger context.

The first known scientific account relating consciousness to the brain dates back to Hippocrates in the fifth century B.C.[1] At that time, there was no formal science as it is recognized today. Hippocrates was nonetheless an acute medical observer and noticed that people with brain damage tended to lose their mental abilities. He realized that mind is something created by the brain and that it dies piece by piece as the brain dies. A passage attributed to him summarizes his view elegantly:

> Men ought to know that from the brain, and from the brain only, arise our pleasures, joys, laughter and jests, as well as our sorrows, pains, griefs and tears. Through it, in particular, we think, see, hear, and distinguish the ugly from the beautiful, the bad from the good, the pleasant from the unpleasant.[1]

The importance of Hippocrates's insight that the brain is the source of the mind cannot be overstated. It launched two and a half thousand years of neuroscience. As a specific explanation of consciousness, however, one has to admit that the Hippocratic account is not very helpful. Rather than explain consciousness, the account merely points to a magician. The brain makes it happen. How the brain does it, and what exactly consciousness may be, Hippocrates left unaddressed. Such questions went beyond the scope of his medical observations.

Two thousand years after Hippocrates, in 1641, Descartes[2] proposed a second influential view of the brain basis of consciousness. In Descartes's view, the mind was made out of an ethereal substance, a fluid, that was stored in a receptacle in the brain. He called the fluid *res cogitans*. Mental substance. When he dissected the brain looking for the receptacle of the soul, he noticed that almost every brain structure came in pairs, one on each side. In his view, the human soul was a single, unified entity, and therefore it could not possibly be divided up and stored in two places. In the end he found a small single lump at the center of the brain, the pineal body, and deduced that it must be the house of the soul. The pineal body is now known to be a gland that produces melatonin and has nothing whatsoever to do with a soul.

Descartes' idea, though refreshingly clever for the time, and though influential in philosophy and theology, did not advance the scientific understanding of consciousness. Instead of proposing an explanation of consciousness, he attributed consciousness to a magic fluid. By what mechanism a fluid substance can cause the experience of consciousness, or where the fluid itself comes from, Descartes left unexplained— truly a case of pointing to a magician instead of explaining the trick.

One of the foundation bricks of modern science, especially modern psychology, is a brilliant treatise so hefty that it is literally rather brick-like, Kant's *A Critique of Pure Reason*, published in 1781.[3] In Kant's account, the mind relies on what he termed "a priori forms," abilities and ideas within us that are present first before all explanations and from which everything else follows. On the subject of consciousness, therefore, Kant had a clear answer: there is no explaining the magic. It is simply supplied to us by divine act. Quite literally, the magician did it.

Hippocrates, Descartes, and Kant represent only three particularly prominent accounts of the mind from the history of science. I could go on describing one famous account after the next and yet get no closer to insight. Even if we fast-forward to modern neuroscience and examine the many proposed theories of consciousness, almost all of them suffer from the same limitation. They are not truly explanatory theories. They point to a magician but do not explain the magic.

One of the first, groundbreaking neurobiological theories of consciousness was proposed in 1990 by the scientists Francis Crick (the co-discoverer of the structure of DNA) and Christof Koch.[4] They suggested that when the electrical signals in the brain oscillate they cause consciousness. The idea, which I will discuss in greater detail later in the book, goes something like this: the brain is composed of neurons that pass information among each other. Information is more efficiently linked from one neuron to another, and more efficiently maintained over short periods of time, if the electrical signals of neurons oscillate in synchrony. Therefore, consciousness might be caused by the electrical activity of many neurons oscillating together.

This theory has some plausibility. Maybe neuronal oscillations are a precondition for consciousness. But note that, once again, the hypothesis is not truly an explanation of consciousness. It identifies a magician. Like the Hippocratic account, "The brain does it" (which is probably true), or like Descartes's account, "The magic fluid inside the brain does it" (which is probably false), this modern theory stipulates that "the oscillations in the brain do it." We still don't know how. Suppose that neuronal oscillations do actually enhance the reliability of information processing. That is impressive and on recent evidence apparently likely to be true.[5-7] But by what logic does that enhanced information processing cause the inner experience? Why an inner feeling? Why should information in the brain—no matter how much its signal strength is boosted, improved, maintained, or integrated from brain site to brain site—become associated with any subjective experience at all? Why is it not just information without the add-on of awareness?

For this type of reason, many thinkers are pessimistic about ever finding an explanation of consciousness. The philosopher Chalmers, in 1995, put it in a way that has become particularly popular.[8] He suggested that the challenge of explaining consciousness can be divided into two problems. One, the easy problem, is to explain how the brain computes and stores information. Calling this problem easy is, of course, a euphemism. What is meant is something more like the technically *possible* problem given a lot of scientific work. In contrast, the hard problem is to explain how we become *aware* of all that stuff going on in the brain. Awareness itself, the essence of awareness, because it is presumed to be nonphysical, because it is by definition private, seems to be scientifically unapproachable. Again, calling it the hard problem is a euphemism; it is the *impossible* problem. We have no choice but to accept it as a mystery. In the hard-problem view, rather than try to explain consciousness, we should marvel at its insolubility.

The hard-problem view has a pinch of defeatism in it. I suspect that for some people it also has a pinch of religiosity. It is a keep-your-scientific-hands-off-my-mystery perspective. One conceptual difficulty with the hard-problem view is that it argues against any explanation of consciousness without knowing what explanations might arise. It is difficult to make a cogent argument against the unknown. Perhaps an explanation exists such that, once we see what it is, once we understand it, we will find that it makes sense and accounts for consciousness.

The current scientific study of consciousness reminds me in many ways of the scientific blind alleys in understanding biological evolution.[9] Charles Darwin published his book *The Origin of Species* in 1859,[10] but long before Darwin, naturalists had already suspected that one species of animal could evolve into another and that different species might be related in a family tree. The idea of a family tree was articulated a century before Darwin, by Linnaeus, in 1758.[11] What was missing, however, was the trick. How was it done? How did various species change over time to become different from each other and to become sophisticated at doing what they needed to do? Scholars explored a few conceptual blind alleys, but a plausible explanation could not be found. Since nobody could think of a mechanistic explanation, since a mechanistic explanation was outside the realm of human imagination, since the richness and complexity of life was obviously too magical for a mundane account, a deity had to be responsible. The magician made it happen. One should accept the grand mystery and not try too hard to explain it.

Then Darwin discovered the trick. A living thing has many off-spring; the offspring vary randomly among each other; and the natural environment, being a harsh place, allows only a select few of those off-spring to procreate, passing on their winning attributes to future generations. Over geological expanses of time, increment by increment, species can undergo extreme changes. Evolution by natural selection. Once you see the trick behind the magic, the insight is so simple as to be either distressing or marvelous, depending on your mood. As

Huxley famously put it in a letter to Darwin, "How stupid of me not to have thought of that!"[12]

The neuroscience of consciousness is, one could say, pre-Darwinian. We are pretty sure the brain does it, but the trick is unknown. Will science find a workable theory of the phenomenon of consciousness?

In this book I propose a theory of consciousness that I hope is unlike most previous theories. This one does not merely point to a magician. It does not merely point to a brain structure or to a brain process and claim without further explanation, *ergo consciousness.* Although I do point to specific brain areas, and although I do point to a specific category of information processed in a specific manner, I also attempt to explain the trick itself. What I am trying to articulate in this book is not just, "Here's the magician that does it," but also, "Here's *how* the magician does it."

For more than twenty years I studied how vision and touch and hearing are combined in the brain and how that information might be used to coordinate the movement of the limbs. I summarized much of that work in a previous book, *The Intelligent Movement Machine,* in 2008.[13] These scientific issues may seem far from the topic of con-sciousness, but over the years I began to realize that basic insights about the brain, about sensory processing and movement control, provided a potential answer to the question of consciousness.

The brain does two things that are of particular importance to the present theory. First, the brain uses a method that most neuroscien-tists call attention. Lacking the resources to processes everything at the same time, the brain focuses its processing on a very few items at any one time. Attention is a data-handling trick for deeply processing some information at the expense of most information. Second, the brain uses internal data to construct simplified, schematic models of objects and events in the world. Those models can be used to make predictions, try out simulations, and plan actions.

What happens when the brain inevitably combines those two talents? In the theory outlined in this book, awareness is the brain's simplified, schematic model of the complicated, data-handling process of attention. Moreover, a brain can use the construct of awareness to model its own attentional state or to model someone else's attentional state. For example, Harry might be focusing his attention on a coffee stain on his shirt. You look at him and understand that Harry is *aware* of the stain. In the theory, much of the same machinery, the same brain regions and computational processing that are used in a social context to attribute awareness to someone else, are also used on a continuous basis to construct your own awareness and attribute it to yourself. Social perception and awareness share a substrate. How that central, simple hypothesis can account for awareness is the topic of this book. The attention schema theory, as I eventually called it, takes a shot at explaining consciousness in a scientifically plausible manner without trivializing the problem.

The theory took rough shape in my mind (in my consciousness, let's say) over a period of about ten years. I eventually outlined it in a chapter of a book for the general public, *God, Soul, Mind, Brain,* published in 2010,[14] and then in a stand-alone neuroscience article that I wrote with Sabine Kastner in 2011.[15] When that article was published, the reaction convinced me that nothing, absolutely nothing about this theory of consciousness was obvious to the rest of the world.

A great many reaction pieces were published by experts on the topic of mind and consciousness and a great many more unpublished commentaries were communicated to me. Many of the commentaries were enthusiastic, some were cautious, and a few were in direct opposition. I am grateful for the feedback, which helped me to further shape the ideas and their presentation. It is always difficult to communicate a new idea. It can take years for the scientific community to figure out what you are talking about, and just as many years for you to figure out how best to articulate the idea. The commentaries, whether friendly or otherwise, convinced me beyond any doubt that a short article was nowhere near sufficient to lay out the theory. I needed to write a book.

The present book is written both for my scientific colleagues and for the interested public. I have tried to be as clear as possible, explaining my terms, assuming no technical knowledge on the part of the reader. To the neuroscientists and cognitive psychologists, I apologize if my explanations are more colloquial than is typical in academia. I was more concerned with explaining concepts than with presenting detail. To the nonexperts, I apologize if the descriptions are sometimes a little wonkish, especially in the second half of the book. I tried to strike a balance.

My purpose in this book is to explain the new theory in a step-by-step manner, to lay out some of the evidence that supports it, and to point out the gaps where the evidence is ambiguous or has yet to come in. Especially on the topic of consciousness, I've discovered how easy it is for people to half-listen to an idea, pigeonhole it, and thereby conveniently dismiss it. My task in this book is to try to explain the theory clearly enough that I can communicate at least some of what it has to offer.

None of us knows for certain how the brain produces consciousness, but the attention schema theory looks promising. It explains the main phenomena. It is logical, conceptually simple, testable, and already has support from a range of previous experiments. I do not put the theory in opposition to the three or four other major neuroscientific views of consciousness. Rather, my approach fuses many previous theories and lines of thought, building a single conceptual framework, combining strengths. For all of these reasons, I am enthusiastic about the theory as a biological explanation of the mind—of consciousness itself—and I am eager to communicate the theory properly.

2

Introducing the Theory

Explaining the attention schema theory is not difficult. Explaining why it is a good theory, and how it meshes with existing evidence, is much more difficult. In this chapter I provide an overview of the theory, acknowledging that the overview by itself is unlikely to convince many people. The purpose of the chapter is to set out the ideas that will be elaborated throughout the remainder of the book.

One way to approach the theory is through social perception. If you notice Harry paying attention to the coffee stain on his shirt, when you see the direction of Harry's gaze, the expression on his face, and his gestures as he touches the stain, and when you put all those clues into context your brain does something quite specific: it attributes awareness to Harry. Harry is aware of the stain on his shirt. Machinery in your brain, in the circuitry that participates in social perception, is expert at this task of attributing awareness to other people. It sees another brain-controlled creature focusing its computing resources on an item and generates the construct that person Y is aware of thing X. In the theory proposed in this book, the same machinery is engaged in attributing awareness to yourself—in computing that you are aware of thing X.

A specific network of brain areas in the cerebral cortex is especially active during social thinking, when people engage with other people and construct ideas about other people's minds. Two brain regions in particular tend to crop up repeatedly in experiments on social thinking. These regions are called the superior temporal sulcus (STS) and the temporo-parietal junction (TPJ). I will have more to say about these brain areas throughout the book. When these regions of the cerebral cortex are damaged, people can suffer from a catastrophic disruption of awareness. The clinical syndrome is called neglect. It is a loss of awareness of objects on one side of space. While it can be caused by damage to a variety of brain areas, it turns out to be especially complete and long-lasting after damage to the TPJ or STS on the right side of the brain.[1,2]

Why should a person lose a part of his or her own awareness after damage to a part of the social machinery? The result is sometimes viewed as contradictory or controversial. But a simple explanation might work here. Maybe the same machinery responsible for attributing awareness to other people also participates in constructing one's own awareness and attributing it to oneself. Just as you can compute that Harry is aware of something, so too you can compute that you yourself are aware of something. The theory proposed in this book was first described from this perspective of social neuroscience.[3,4]

Theories of consciousness, because they are effectively theories of the soul, tend to have far-reaching cultural, spiritual, and personal implications. If consciousness is a construct of the social machinery, if this social machinery attributes awareness to others and to oneself, then perhaps a great range of attributed conscious minds—gods, angels, devils, spirits, ghosts, the consciousness we attribute to pets, to other people, and the consciousness we confidently attribute to ourselves—are manifestations of the same underlying process. The spirit world and its varied denizens may be constructs of the social machinery in the human brain, models of minds attributed to the objects and spaces around us.

In this book I will touch on all of these topics, from the science of specific brain areas to the more philosophical questions of mind and spirit. The emphasis of the book, however, is on the theory itself—the attention schema theory of how a brain produces awareness. The purpose of this chapter is to provide an initial description of the theory.

Consciousness and Awareness

One of the biggest obstacles to discussing consciousness is the great many definitions of it. I find that conversations go in circles because of terminological confusion. The first order of business is to define my use of two key terms. In my experience, people have personal, quirky definitions of the term *consciousness*, whereas everyone more or less agrees on the meaning of the term *awareness*. In this section, for clarity, I draw a distinction between consciousness and awareness. Many such distinctions have been made in the past, and here I describe one way to parcel out the concepts.

Figure 2.1 diagrams the proposed relationship between the terms. The scheme has two components. The first component is the information about which I am aware. I am aware of the room around me, the sound of traffic from the street outside, my own body, my own thoughts and emotions, the memories brought up in my mind at the moment. All of these items are encoded in my brain as chunks of information. I am aware of a great diversity of information. The second component shown in the diagram is the act of being aware of the information. That, of course, is the mystery. Not all information

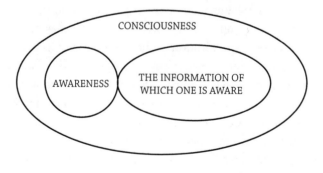

FIGURE 2.1

One way to define consciousness and awareness. Consciousness is inclusive, and awareness is a specific act applied to the information that is in consciousness.

in the brain has awareness attached to it. Indeed, most of it does not. Some extra thing or process must be required to make me aware of a specific chunk of information in my brain at a particular time.

As shown in the same diagram, I use the term *consciousness* inclusively. It refers both to the information about which I am aware and to the process of being aware of it. In this scheme, *consciousness* is the more general term and *awareness* the more specific. Consciousness encompasses the whole of personal experience at any moment, whereas awareness applies only to one part, the act of experiencing. I acknowledge, however, that other people may have alternative definitions.

I hope the present definitions will help to avoid certain types of confusion. For example, some thinkers have insisted to me, "To explain consciousness, you must explain how I experience color, touch, temperature, the raw sensory feel of the world." Others have insisted, "To explain consciousness, you must explain how I know who I am, how I know that I am here, how I know that I am a person distinct from the rest of the world." Yet others have said, "To explain consciousness, you must explain memory, because calling up memories gives me my self-identity."

Each of these suggestions involves an awareness of a specific type of knowledge. Explaining self-knowledge, for example, is in principle easy. A computer also "knows" what it is. It has an information file on its own specifications. It has a memory of its prior states. Self-knowledge is merely another category of knowledge. How knowledge can be encoded in the brain is not fundamentally mysterious, but how we become *aware* of the information is. Whether I am aware of myself as a person, or aware of the feel of a cool breeze, or aware of a color, or aware of an emotion, the awareness itself is the mystery to be explained, not the specific knowledge about which I am aware.

The purpose of this book is not to explain the content of consciousness. It is not to explain the knowledge that generally composes consciousness. It is not to explain memories or self-understanding or emotion or vision or touch. The purpose of the book is to present a theory of awareness. How can we become aware of any information at all? What is added to produce awareness? I will argue that the added ingredient is, itself, information. It is information of a specific type that serves a specific function. The following sections begin with the relationship between awareness and information, and gradually build to the attention schema theory.

A Squirrel in the Head

In this section, I use an unusual example to illustrate the idea that awareness might be information instantiated in the brain.

I had a friend who was a clinical psychologist. He once told me about a patient of his. The patient was delusional and thought that he had a squirrel inside his head. He was certain of it. No argument could convince him otherwise. He might agree that the condition was physically impossible or illogical, but his squirrelness transcended physics or logic. You could ask him why he was so convinced, and he would report that the squirrel had nothing to do with him being convinced or not. You could ask him if he felt fur and claws on the inside of his skull, and he would say, although the squirrel did have fur and claws, his belief had nothing to do with sensing those features. The squirrel was simply there. He knew it. He had direct access to his squirrelness. Instead of Descartes's famous phrase, "Cogito ergo sum," this man's slogan could have been, "Squirrel ergo squirrel." Or, to be technical, "Sciurida ergo sciurida."

The squirrel in the man's head poses two intellectual problems. We might call them the easy problem and the hard problem.

The easy problem is to figure out how a brain might arrive at that conclusion with such certainty. The brain is an information-processing device. Not all the information available to it and not all its internal processes are perfect. When a person introspects, his or her brain is accessing internal data. If the internal data is wrong or unrealistic, the brain will arrive at a wrong or unrealistic conclusion. Not only might the conclusion be wrong, but the brain might incorrectly assign a high degree of certainty to it. Level of certainty is after all a computation that, like all computations, can go awry. People have been known to be dead certain of patently ridiculous and false information. All of these errors in computation are understandable, at least in general terms. The man's brain had evidently constructed a description of a squirrel in his head, complete with bushy tail, claws, and beady eyes. His cognitive machinery accessed that description, incorrectly assigned a high certainty of reality to it, and reported it. So much for the easy problem.

But then there is the hard problem. How can a brain, a mere assemblage of neurons, result in an actual squirrel inside the man's head? How is the squirrel produced? Where does the fur come from? Where do the claws, the tail, and the beady little eyes come from? How does all that rich complex squirrel stuff emerge? Now that is a very hard problem indeed. It seems physically impossible. No known process can lead from neuronal circuitry to squirrel. What is the magic?

If we all shared that man's delusion, if it were a ubiquitous fixture of the human brain, if it were evolutionarily built into us, we would be scientifically stumped by that hard problem. We would introspect, find the squirrel in us with all its special properties, be certain of its existence, describe it to each other, and agree collectively that we each have it. And yet we would have no idea how to explain the jump from neuronal circuitry to squirrel. We would have no idea how to explain the mysterious disappearance of the squirrel on autopsy. Confronted with a philosophical, existential conundrum, we would be forced into the dualist position that the brain is somehow both a neuronal machine and, at the same time, on a higher plane, a squirrel.

Of course, there is no hard problem because there is no actual squirrel. The man's brain contains a description of a squirrel, not an actual squirrel. When you consider it, an actual squirrel would be an extremely poor explanation for his beliefs and behavior. There is no obvious mechanism to get from a squirrel somehow inserted into his head to his decision, belief, certainty, insistence, and report about it. Postulating that there is an actual squirrel does not help explain anything. I suppose in a philosophical sense you could say the squirrel exists, but it exists as information. It exists as a description.

I suggest that when the word *squirrel* is replaced with the word *awareness*, the logic remains the same. We think it is inside us. We have direct access to it. We are certain we have it. We agree on its basic properties. But where does the inner feeling come from? How can neurons possibly create it? How can we explain the jump from physical brain to ethereal awareness? How can we solve the hard problem?

The answer may be that there is no hard problem. The properties of conscious experience—the tail, claws, and eyeballs of it so to speak; the feeling, the vividness, the raw *experienceness*, and the ethereal nature of it, its ghostly presence inside our bodies and especially inside our heads— these properties may be explainable as components of a descriptive model. The brain does not contain these things: it contains a *description* of these things. Brains are good at constructing descriptions of things. At least in principle it is easy to understand how a brain might construct information, how it might construct a detailed, rich description of having a conscious experience, of possessing awareness, how it might assign a high degree of certainty to that described state, and how it might scan that information and thereby insist that it has that state.

In the case of the man who thought he had a squirrel in his head, one can dismiss his certainty as a delusion. The delusion serves no adaptive function. It is harmful. It impedes normal everyday functioning. Thank goodness few of us have that delusion. I am decidedly *not* suggesting that awareness is a delusion. In the attention schema theory, awareness is not a harmful error but instead an adaptive, useful, internal model. But like the squirrel in the head, it is a *description* of a thing, not the thing itself. The challenge of the theory is to explain why a brain should expend the energy on constructing such an elaborate description. What is its use? Why construct information that describes such a particular collection of properties? Why an inner essence? Why an inner feeling? Why that specific ethe-real relationship between me and a thing of which I am aware? If the brain is to construct descriptions of itself, why construct that idiosyncratic one, and why is it so efficacious as to be ready-built into the brains of almost all people? The attention schema theory is a proposed answer to those questions.

Arrow B

Figure 2.2 shows one way to depict the relationship between con-sciousness and the brain. Almost all scientific work on conscious-ness focuses on Arrow A: how does the brain produce an awareness

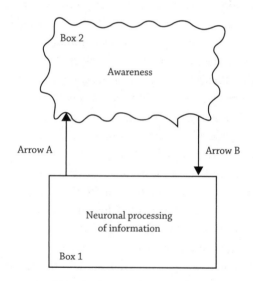

FIGURE 2.2

A traditional view in which awareness emerges from the processing of information in the brain (Arrow A). Awareness must also affect the brain's information processing (Arrow B), or we would be unable to say that we are aware.

of something? Granted that the brain processes information, how do we become aware of the information? But any useful theory of consciousness must also deal with Arrow B. Once you have an awareness of something, how does the feeling itself impact the neuronal machinery, such that the presence of awareness can be reported?

One of the only truths about awareness that we can know with objective certainty is that we can say that we have it. Of course, we don't report all our conscious experiences. Some are probably unreportable. Language is a limited medium. But because we can, at least sometimes, say that we are aware of this or that, we can learn something about awareness itself. Speech is a physical, measurable act. It is caused by the action of muscles, which are controlled by neurons, which operate by manipulation and transmission of information. Whatever awareness is, it must be able to physically impact neuronal signals. Otherwise we would be unable to say that we have it and I would not be writing this book.

It is with Arrow B that many of the common notions of awareness fail. It is one thing to theorize about Arrow A, about how the functioning of the brain might result in awareness. But if your theory lacks an Arrow B, if it fails to explain how the emergent awareness can physically cause specific signals in specific neurons, such that speech can occur, then your theory fails to explain the one known objective property of awareness: we can at least sometimes say that we have it. Most theories of consciousness are magical in two ways. First, Arrow A is magical. How awareness emerges from the brain is unexplained. Second, Arrow B is magical. How awareness controls the brain is unexplained.

This problem of double magic disappears if awareness is information. The brain is, after all, an information-processing device. For an information-processing device to report that it has inner, subjective experience, it must contain within it information to that effect. The cognitive machinery can then access that information, read it, summarize it linguistically, and provide a verbal report to the outside world.

One of the nice properties of a description is that almost anything can be described, even things that are physically impossible or logically inconsistent or magical. Such as Gandalf the Wizard. Or Escher-like infinite staircases. Or a squirrel in the head. Such things can be painted in as much nuanced detail as one likes in the form of information. Even if these things don't exist as such, they can be described. If awareness is *described* by the brain rather than *produced* by the brain, then explaining its properties becomes considerably easier.

Suppose that you are looking at a green object and have a conscious experience of greenness. In the view that I am suggesting, the brain contains a chunk of information that describes the state of experiencing, and it contains a chunk of information that describes spectral green. Those two chunks are bound together. In that way, the brain computes a larger, composite description of experiencing green. Once that description is in place, other machinery accesses the description, abstracts information from it, summarizes it, and can verbalize it. The brain can, after all, report only the information that it has. This approach to consciousness is depicted schematically in Figure 2.3.

This approach is deeply unsatisfying—which does not argue against it. A theory does not need to be satisfying to be true. The approach is unsatisfying partly because it takes away some of the magic. It says, in effect, there is no subjective feeling inside, at least not quite as people

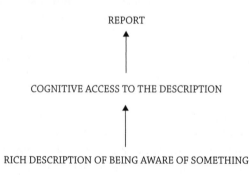

FIGURE 2.3

Awareness as information instantiated in the brain. Access to the information allows us to say that we are aware.

have typically imagined it. Instead, there is a description of having a feeling and a computed certainty that the description is accurate and not merely a description. The brain, accessing that information, can then act in the ways that we know people to act—it can decide that it has a subjective feeling, and it can talk about the subjective feeling.

The Awareness Feature

Let's explore further what it might mean for awareness to be a description constructed by circuitry in the brain. The brain is an expert at constructing descriptions. When you look at an apple, your visual system encodes and combines many sensory features. Some of these features are diagrammed in Figure 2.4. Perhaps the apple is green. It's more or less round. Perhaps it's moving—rolling to the right. Binding of stimulus features such as color and shape and motion into a single larger representation has been studied intensively, especially in the domain of visual perception.[5]

I am suggesting that the property of awareness is another such computed feature, a description, a chunk of information, that can be bound to the larger object file. The many chunks of information

GREEN + ROUND + MOTION + AWARENESS

FIGURE 2.4

Awareness as a computed feature. A green apple is encoded in the visual system as a set of stimulus features described by chunks of information that are bound together. The property of awareness might be another computed stimulus feature bound to the rest.

depicted in Figure 2.4 are connected into a single representation, a description in which the greenness, the roundness, the movement, and the property of having a conscious experience, are wedded together. My cognitive machinery can access that information, that bound representation, and report on it. Hence the machinery of my brain can report that it is aware of the apple and its features.

In this account, awareness is information; it is a description; it is a description of the experiencing of something; and it is a perception-like feature, in the sense that it can be bound to other features to help form an overarching description of an object.

I suggest that there is no other way for an information-processing device, such as a brain, to conclude that it has a conscious experience attached to an apple. It must construct an informational description of the apple, an informational description of conscious experience, and bind the two together.

The object does not need to be an apple, of course. The explanation is potentially general. Instead of visual information about an apple you could have touch information, or a representation of a math equation, or a representation of an emotion, or a representation of your own personhood, or a representation of the words you are reading at this moment. Awareness, as a chunk of information, could in principle be bound to any of these other categories of information. Hence you could be aware of the objects around you, of sights and sounds, of introspective content, of your physical body, of your emotional state, of your own personal identity. You could bind the awareness feature to many different types of information.

Why would the brain construct such a strange chunk of information unless it represents something of use in the real world?

The brain constructs descriptions of real entities in the real world. Those descriptions may not always be accurate. They may be simplified or schematized, but they generally reflect something useful to know. When the brain encodes information about the color of an apple, for example, that information relates to something physically real—wavelengths reflecting from the surface of the apple. What real or useful property might be represented by this strange chunk of information that describes the state of being aware? Why attach an "awareness feature" to the other, more concrete features in order to make up the brain's description of an apple?

The theory can be put in a sentence: Awareness is a description of attention.

Awareness as a Sketch of Attention

When people use the word *attention* colloquially, it has a variety of meanings. Are you paying attention to my book? The guy in the next office is an attention seeker. Attention all shoppers! The term is also used scientifically. In cognitive psychology, it refers to an enhanced way of reacting to incoming stimuli. In neuroscience, it refers to a type of interaction among signals in the brain. I am going to give you a neuroscientist's perspective: attention as a data-handling method in the brain. From now on, when I use the term *attention*, I will mean it in this technical, neuroscience sense.

In Figure 2.5, the circles represent competing signals in the brain. These signals are something like political candidates in an election. Each signal works to win a stronger voice and suppress its neighbors. Attention is when one integrated set of signals rises in strength and outcompetes other signals. Each signal can gain a boost from a variety of sources. Strong sensory input, coming from the outside, can boost a particular signal in the brain (a bottom-up bias), or a high-level decision in the brain can boost a particular signal (a top-down bias). As a winning signal emerges and suppresses competing signals, as it shouts louder and causes the competition to hush, it gains a larger influence over other processing in the brain and, therefore, over behavior. Attending to an apple means that the neuronal representation of the apple grows stronger, wins the competition of the moment, and suppresses the representations of

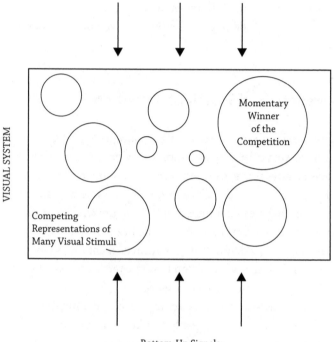

FIGURE 2.5

Attention as a data-handling method. Here visual attention is illustrated. Visual stimuli are represented by patterns of activity in the visual system. The many representations in the visual system are in constant competition. At any moment, one representation wins the competition, gains in signal strength, and suppresses other representations. The winning representation tends to dominate processing in the brain and thus behavior. A similar data-handling method is thought to occur in other brain systems outside the visual system.

other stimuli. The apple representation can then more easily influence behavior. This description of attention is based on an account worked out by Desimone and colleagues, called the "biased competition model of attention."[6-8] It also has some similarity to a classic account proposed by Selfridge in the 1950s called the "pandemonium model."[9]

Attention is not data encoded in the brain; it is a data-handling method. It is an act. It is something the brain does, a procedure, an emergent process. Signals compete with each other and a winner emerges—like bubbles rising up out of water. As circumstances shift, a new winner emerges. There is no reason for the brain to have any explicit knowledge about the process or dynamics of attention. Water boils but has no knowledge of how it does it. A car can move but has no knowledge of how it does it. I am suggesting, however, that in addition to *doing* attention, the brain also constructs a *description* of attention, a quick sketch of it so to speak, and awareness is that description.

A schema is a coherent set of information that, in a simplified but useful way, represents something more complex. In the present theory, awareness is an attention schema. It is not attention but rather a simplified, useful description of attention. Awareness allows the brain to understand attention, its dynamics, and its consequences.

Consider the apple in Figure 2.4. The brain constructs chunks of information to describe the color of the apple, the shape of the apple, and the motion of the apple. These features are bound together to form a larger description of the apple. According to the present theory, the brain also constructs a chunk of information to describe one's own attention being focused on the apple.

In this theory, awareness is handled by the brain like color. Awareness and color are computed features. They are representations. They represent something physically real—wavelength in the case of color, attention in the case of awareness.

The awareness feature can be bound to color and to many other features as the brain constructs an overarching representation of an object. If the object is a green apple, its representation in the brain could be diagrammed as $V + A$, where V stands for visual features (roundness, greenness, movement) and A stands for the chunk of information that depicts awareness. Cognitive access to that bound description allows the brain to conclude and report not only that the object has this shape and that color, this motion and that location, but that these properties come with awareness fused to them.

If the hypothesis is correct, if awareness is a schema that describes attention, then we should be able to find similarities between awareness and attention. These similarities have been noted before by many scientists.[10-13] Here I am suggesting a specific reason why awareness and attention are so similar to each other: the one is the brain's schematic description of the other. Awareness is a sketch of attention. Below I list eight key similarities.

1. Both involve a target. You attend *to* something. You are aware *of* something.
2. Both involve an agent. Attention is performed by a brain. Awareness implies an "I" who is aware.
3. Both are selective. Only a small fraction of available information is attended at any one time. Awareness is selective in the same way. You are aware of only a tiny amount of the information impinging on your senses at any one time.
4. Both are graded. Attention typically has a single focus, but while attending mostly to A, the brain spares some attention for B. Awareness also has a focus and is graded in the same manner. One can be most intently aware of A and a little aware of B.
5. Both operate on similar domains of information. Although most studies of attention focus on vision, it is certainly not limited to vision. The same signal enhancement can be applied to any of the five senses, to a thought, to an emotion, to a recalled memory, or to a plan to make a movement, for example. Likewise, one can be aware of the same range of items. If you can attend to it, then you can be aware of it.

6. Both imply an effect on behavior. When the brain attends to something, the neural signals are enhanced, gain greater influence over the downstream circuitry, and have a greater impact on behavior. When the brain does not attend to something, the neural representation is weak and has relatively little impact on behavior. Likewise, when you are aware of something, you can choose to act on it. When you are unaware of something, you will generally fail to react to it. Both, therefore, imply an ability to drive behavior.

7. Both imply deep processing. Attention is when an information processor devotes computing resources to an information set. Awareness implies an intelligence seizing on, being occupied by, experiencing, or knowing something.

8. Finally, and particularly tellingly, awareness almost always tracks attention. Awareness is like a needle on a dial pointing more or less to the state of one's attention. At any moment in time, the information that is attended usually matches the information that reaches awareness. In some situations they can be separated.[10,11,14–16] It is possible to attend to a visual image by all behavioral measures, processing the picture in depth and even responding to it, while being unaware of it. Because attention and awareness can be dissociated, we know that they are not the same thing. But mismatches between them are rare. Awareness is evidently a close but imperfect indicator of attention.

Many more comparisons are possible, but I have listed at least the main ones. The point of the list is that awareness can be understood as an imperfect but close model of attention.

Consider how the brain models the property of color, in particular the color white. White light contains a mixture of all wavelengths in the visible spectrum. It is the dirtiest, muddiest color possible. But the visual system does not model it in that way. Instead, the visual system encodes the information of high brightness and low color. That is the brain's model of white light—a high value of brightness and a low value of color, a purity of luminance—a physical impossibility. Why does the brain construct a physically impossible description of a part of the world? The purpose of that inner model is not to be physically accurate in all details, which would be a waste of neural processing. Instead, the purpose is to provide a quick sketch, a representation that is easy to compute, convenient, and just accurate enough to be useful in guiding behavior.

By the same token, in the present hypothesis, the brain constructs a model of the attentional process. That model involves some physically nonsensical properties: an ethereal thing like plasma vaguely localizable to the space inside us, an experience that is intangible, a feeling that has no physicality. Here I am proposing that those nonphysical properties and other common properties ascribed to awareness are schematic, approximate descriptions of a real physical process. The physical process being modeled is something mechanistic and complicated and neuronal, a process of signal enhancement, the process of attention. When cognitive machinery scans and summarizes internal data, it has no direct access to the process of attention itself. Instead, it has access to the data in the attention schema. It can access, summarize, and report the contents of that information set. Introspection returns an answer based on a quick, approximate sketch, a cartoon of attention, the item we call awareness. Awareness is the brain's cartoon of attention.

How Awareness Relates to Other Components of the Conscious Mind

Consider a simple sentence:

I am aware of X.

Pick any X you like. An apple. A sound. The thought 2 + 2 = 4. The emotion of joy. I am aware of X. To be able to report this, and actually mean it, my brain must possess three chunks of information all bound together:

$$[I] \ [\text{am aware of}] \ [X].$$

In pursuing consciousness, one possible approach is to focus on the first part, the knowledge of the self, the "I" in "I am aware of X." One aspect of self-knowledge is body knowledge. The "body schema" is a rich understanding of your physical self, of the distinction between physical objects that belong to your personhood (this is my hand, this is my leg) and objects that are outside of you (this is somebody else's hand, this is the chair). A second aspect of self-knowledge is psychological knowledge. You have knowledge of your own mind, including knowledge about current thoughts and emotions, about autobiographical memories that define your sense of personhood. Your knowledge of self is based on a vast range of information. Does the secret of consciousness lie in this "I" side of the equation? The self-knowledge approach to consciousness, while doing a good job of explaining why we have detailed information about ourselves, does a poor job of explaining how we become aware of that information or of anything else. I will discuss this general approach in much greater detail in Chapter 10.

Another possible approach to consciousness is to focus on the object of the awareness, the "X" in "I am aware of X." The assumption is that, if you are aware of a visual stimulus, then awareness must be created by the visual circuitry. Some trick of the neuronal interactions, some oscillation, some feedback, some vibration causes visual awareness to emerge. Tactile awareness must arise from the circuitry that computes touch. Awareness of emotion must arise from the circuitry that computes emotion. Awareness of an abstract thought might arise from somewhere in the frontal lobe where the thought is presumably computed. Awareness, in that view, is a byproduct of information. Brain circuitry computes X, and an awareness of X rises up from the circuitry like heat. Why we end up with a unified awareness, if every brain region generates its own private awareness, is not clear. It is also not clear how the feeling of awareness itself, having been produced, having risen up from the information, ends up physically impacting the speech circuitry such that we can sometimes report that we have it. I will discuss this approach in greater detail in Chapter 11.

In contrast to these common approaches, in this book I am pointing to an overlooked chunk of information that lies between the "I" and the "X," the information that defines the relationship between them, the proposed attention schema. In the theory proposed here, awareness itself does not arise from the information about which you are aware, and it is not your knowledge that *you*, in particular, are aware of it. It is instead your rich descriptive model of the relationship between an agent and the information being attended by the agent.

The other two components are important. Without them, awareness makes no sense. Without an agent to be aware, and without a thing to be aware of, the middle bit has no use. I do not mean to deny the importance of the other components. They are a part of consciousness. But awareness itself, the essence of awareness, I propose to be specifically the piece in the middle: the attention schema.

Awareness and Social Perception

The attention schema is not so far-fetched a hypothesis. We already know the brain contains something like it. The brain contains specialized machinery that computes a description of someone else's state of attention. It is part of the machinery for social thinking.[17-21]

Humans have an ability to monitor the gaze of others. We know where other people are looking. The scientific work on social attention, as it is sometimes called, has tended to limit itself to detecting someone else's gaze direction.[17,22-24] But I doubt that our sophisticated machinery for understanding other people's attention is limited to vector geometry based on the eyes. Computing where someone else is looking is, in a sense, incidental. Computing someone else's attentional state is a deeper task. I argue that we have a rich, sophisticated model of what attention is, of how it is deployed, of its temporal and spatial dynamics, of its consequences on action. A model of that type is essential to understanding and predicting another person's behavior. Gaze direction is merely one visual cue that can help to inform that model. After all, blind people, with no visual cues about someone else's gaze direction, still understand other people's attention.

As diagrammed in Figure 2.6, the proposed attention schema can *use* gaze direction as a cue, but does not necessarily do so. It brings together a totality of evidence to constrain a rather rich and sophisticated model of someone else's attention. It can use that model to help understand other people and predict their behavior. I am proposing that the same machinery used to model another person's attentional state in a social situation is also used to model one's own attentional state. The benefit is the same: understanding and predicting one's own behavior. The machinery is in this sense general.

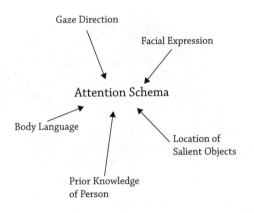

FIGURE 2.6

The attention schema, the hypothesized model of attentional state and attentional dynamics, relies on information from many sources. Diagrammed here are some of the cues from which we reconstruct someone else's attentional state.

Where in the brain should we look for this proposed attention schema? The theory makes three broad predictions about the brain areas involved.

First, a brain system that constructs the attention schema should be active when people engage in social perception. It should be involved in monitoring or reconstructing other people's mind states, especially reconstructing the state of other people's attention.

Second, a brain system that constructs the attention schema should somehow track or reflect a person's own changing state of attention.

Third, when that brain system is damaged or disrupted, awareness itself should be disrupted.

Do any areas of the brain satisfy these predictions? It turns out that all three properties overlap in a region of the cerebral cortex that lies just above the ear, with a relative emphasis on the right side of the brain. Within that brain region, two adjacent areas have been studied most intensively. These areas are shown in Figure 2.7. (A scan of my

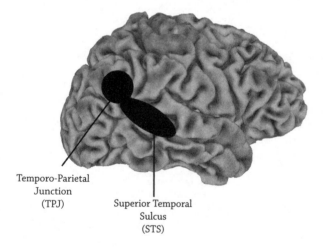

Temporo-Parietal
Junction
(TPJ)

Superior Temporal
Sulcus
(STS)

FIGURE 2.7

Two areas of the human brain that might be relevant to social intelligence.

own right cerebral hemisphere, by the way.) They are the superior temporal sulcus (STS) and the temporo-parietal junction (TPJ). These areas are probably themselves collections of smaller, specialized subunits that presumably work in a cooperative fashion and interact with larger, brain-wide networks. I will describe the details of the TPJ and the STS in later chapters. Here I merely note in brief that they combine the three key properties predicted by the attention schema theory. First, these areas are recruited during social perception. Second, they track one's own state of attention. Third, damage to them leads to a devastating clinical disruption of awareness. Each of these three properties was discovered and studied separately, and the collision of the three properties in one region of the brain has caused some controversy. How can such diverse, seemingly unrelated properties be reconciled? The attention schema theory may help to solve the riddle by fitting the many results into a single framework.

In the present theory, the *content* of consciousness, the stuff *in* the conscious mind, is distributed over a large set of brain areas, areas that encode vision, emotion, language, action plans, and so on. The full set of information that is present in consciousness at any one time has been called the "global workspace."[25,26] In the present theory, the global workspace spans many diverse areas of the brain. But the specific property of awareness, the *essence* of awareness added to the global workspace, is constructed by an expert system in a limited part of the brain, perhaps centered on the TPJ or STS and perhaps involving other brain regions. The computed property of awareness can be bound to the larger whole. As a result, the brain can report that awareness is attached to a color, that awareness is attached to a sound, that awareness is attached to an abstract thought.

This account of consciousness gives an especially simple explanation for why so much information, the majority of processing in the brain, can never reach consciousness. Much of the information in the brain may not be directly linkable to the attention schema. Only brain areas that are appropriately linkable to the attention schema can participate in consciousness.

Even information that can in principle be linked to the attention schema might not always be so. For example, not everything that comes in through the eyes and is processed in the visual system reaches reportable awareness. Not all of our actions are planned and executed with our conscious participation. Systems that can, under some circumstances, function in the purview of awareness at other times seem to function with equal complexity and sophistication in the absence of awareness. In the present theory, the explanation is simply that the information computed by these systems is sometimes linked or bound to the attention schema, and sometimes not. The shifting coalitions in the brain determine what information is bound to the attention schema and thus included in consciousness, and what information is not bound to the attention schema and thus operating outside of consciousness.

This account of consciousness is easily misunderstood. I will take a moment here to point out what I am *not* saying. I am not saying that a central area of the brain lurking inside us is aware of this and that. It is tempting to go the homunculus route—the little-man-in-the-head route—to postulate that some central area of the brain is aware, and that it is aware of information supplied to it by other brain regions. This version, a little man aware of what the rest of the brain is telling him, is entirely nonexplanatory; it is a variant of "the magician does it."

Instead, according to the present theory, awareness is a constructed feature. It is a complex chunk of descriptive information, A. It can be linked to other information. For example, information A may be linked to information X, constructing a larger, brain-spanning chunk of information, $A + X$. When you report that you are aware of X—that X comes with the property of awareness associated with it—it is because your cognitive machinery has accessed that larger chunk of information, $A + X$, and summarized its contents.

Visual information is obviously required for visual consciousness. Touch information is necessary for tactile awareness. The information that $2 + 2 = 4$ is obviously necessary to be aware of the abstract thought $2 + 2 = 4$. Sets of information about oneself, one's own thoughts and emotions and memories, are required to understand who, exactly, is conscious. All of these chunks of information are part of a normal state of consciousness. By themselves, however, they are merely representations of things. Representations of objects. Representations of thoughts and emotions. Representations of a physical body. It is hard to understand how cognition could scan such a pile of representations and report the presence of awareness. A brain would be able to report this is green, that is big, my elbow is bent, $2 + 2 = 4$, I ate ice cream yesterday, but not that it consciously experiences any of that material. It would be silent on the topic of consciousness. But with a schematic description of attention bound to the larger set, with the attention schema, cognition can scan the available information and on that basis conclude that awareness is present—not only that X is so, but that I am aware of X. With that we have an account of where consciousness comes from, what it is, what its adaptive value is, how we introspect about it, and how we report on it.

Again, I would like to be clear on what the theory does *not* explain. You cannot get from the attention schema theory to the construction of an actual, ethereal, ectoplasmic, nonphysical, inner feeling. Like the case of the squirrel in the head, the brain constructs a *description* of inner experience, not the item itself. The construction of an actual inner experience as we intuitively understand it, as we note it in ourselves, as we describe it to each other is not necessary. Whatever we are talking about when we talk about consciousness, it can't be that, because the feeling wouldn't have any route to get into our speech. The conclusions, certainties, reports, and eloquent poetry spoken about it all require information as a basis. To explain the behavior of the machine we need *the data set that describes awareness*. The awareness itself is out of the loop.

Strange Loops

I hardly want readers to get the impression that the attention schema theory is tidy. When you think about its implementation in the brain, it quickly becomes strange in ways that may begin to resemble actual human experience. This final section of the chapter summarizes one of the stranger complexities of the theory. I will discuss more complexities in later chapters.

If the theory is correct, then awareness is a description, a representation, constructed in the brain. The thing being represented is attention. But attention is the process of enhancing representations in the brain. We have a strange loop—a snake eating its own tail, or a hand drawing itself, so to speak. (Hofstadter coined the term "strange loop" in his 1979 book *Godel, Escher, Bach*[27] and suggested that some type of strange loop might be at the root of consciousness.) In the present theory, awareness is a representation of the process that enhances representations. If that account is correct, then being aware of something and attending to it feed each other. The two are in a positive feedback loop: they are like two mirrors facing each other. Boost one and you boost the other. Damage one and you deflate the other. Attention cannot work fully without awareness, nor awareness without attention.

Thus far, in summarizing the theory, I have tended to emphasize the distinction between awareness and attention. Attention is an active process, a data-handling style that boosts this or that chunk of information in the brain. In contrast, awareness is a description, a chunk of information, a reflection of the ongoing state of attention. Yet because of the strange loop between awareness and attention, the functions of the two are blurred together. Awareness becomes just as much of an active controller as attention. Awareness helps direct signals in the brain, enhancing some, suppressing others, guiding choices and actions.

The idea of a description that also acts is not new. One common example is the phrase, "I pronounce you husband and wife." The words describe a state of marriage but also cause the state to be true. Another example is the mission statement of a company. It is a description of what the company does, but by providing a handy, memorable slogan, the words also help make the company do it. A third example might be writing a description in your diary of how you feel. The description itself shapes and alters how you feel. Here I am suggesting that the attention schema is a case of a description that helps make it so. Not only does the attention schema provide the brain with a descriptive model of attention, but the description itself must help to direct attention and thereby to direct behavior.

A long-standing question about consciousness is whether it is passive or active. Does it merely observe, or does it also cause? One of the more colorful metaphors on the topic was suggested by the philosopher Haidt.[28] The unconscious machinery of the brain is so vast that it is like an elephant. Perhaps consciousness is a little boy sitting on the elephant's head. The boy naïvely imagines that he is in control of the elephant, but he merely watches what the elephant chooses to do. He is a passive observer with a delusion of control. Alternatively, perhaps consciousness has the reins and is at least partially in control of the elephant. Is awareness solely a passive observer or also an active participant? The present theory comes down on the side of an active participant. Awareness is not merely watching, but plays a role in directing brain function.

Hopefully, this chapter has given a general sense of the theory that awareness is an attention schema, of where that theory is coming from and what it is trying to accomplish. I do not expect such a cursory overview to be convincing, but at least it can set out the basic ideas. In the remainder of the book I will begin all over again, this time introducing the theory more systematically and with greater attention to detail. The first half of the book focuses on describing the theory itself. The second half of the book focuses on the relationship to previous scientific theories of consciousness and to experimental evidence from neuroscience.

At the end of the book I take up what might be called mystical or spiritual questions. Even if consciousness is not eternal ectoplasm, but instead information instantiated in the brain, it is nonetheless all the spirit we have. We should treat the spirit with some respect.

The phenomenon can be explored not only from the point of view of mechanism but also from the point of view of human culture and psychological need. A mechanistic theory of consciousness, far from literalizing the world and shriveling spirituality, might actually lead to greater insight and greater satisfaction in spiritual experience.

3

Awareness as Information

In the previous chapter, introducing a rough outline of the theory, I proposed that awareness is information. The proposal initially sounds unlikely. We all know intuitively what awareness is—it is an inner experience and it does not resemble typed words on a page or the ones and zeros of a computer printout. It does not resemble our culturally accepted metaphors for information. How can awareness itself be information? In this chapter I would like to begin again, more systematically, more thoroughly, investigating what awareness is, what its relationship to information may be, and how a brain might make awareness possible.

To set up the problem, I will begin with a traditional way to think about awareness. Consider again Figure 2.2. When information is processed in the brain in some specific but as yet undetermined way (Box 1), a subjective experience of awareness emerges (Box 2). Suppose that you are looking at a green apple. First, your visual system computes the approximate reflectance spectrum of the apple, at least as filtered through the limited detectors of the eye. The presence of this information in the brain can be measured directly by inserting electrodes into visual areas and monitoring the activity of neurons. Second, as a result of that information, for unknown reasons, you have a conscious experience of greenness. You are, of course, aware of other features of the apple, such as its shape and smell, but for the moment let us focus on the particular conscious sensation of greenness. One could say that two items are relevant to the discussion: the computation that the apple is green (Box 1 in Figure 2.2), and the "experienceness" of the green (Box 2).

Arrow A in Figure 2.2 represents the as-yet unknown process by which the brain generates a conscious experience. Arrow A is the central mystery to which scientists of consciousness have addressed themselves, with no definite answer or common agreement. It is difficult to figure out how a physical machine can produce what is commonly assumed to be a nonphysical feeling. Our inability to conceive of a route from physical process to mental experience is the reason for the persistent tradition of pessimism in the scientific study of consciousness. When Descartes[1] claimed that *res extensa* (the physical substance of the body) can never be used to construct *res cogitans* (mental substance), when Kant[2] indicated that our essential mental abilities simply *are* and have no external explanation, and when Chalmers[3] euphemistically referred to the "hard problem" of consciousness, all of these pessimistic views derive from the sheer human inability to imagine how any Arrow A could possibly get from Box 1 to Box 2.

What I would like to do, however, is to focus on Arrow B, a process that is relatively (though not entirely) ignored both scientifically and philosophically. Arrow B represents the process by which a subjective conscious experience, an awareness of something, can physically impact the information-processing systems of the brain, allowing us to report that we have the feeling of awareness. It is my contention that much more can be learned about awareness by considering Arrow B than by considering Arrow A. By asking what, specifically, awareness can *do* in the world, what it can affect, what it can physically cause, we gain the leverage of objectivity. Instead of losing ourselves in speculation and subjectivity, we can pin the investigation on something that is verifiable. My claim is that by starting with Arrow B, one can work backward and obtain a possible answer to the question. I will begin with the verbal ability to report that we are aware, and from that observation take four steps back into the brain toward the property of awareness itself.

The Report of Awareness

Let's start with the verbal report of awareness. You might say, "The apple is green." But a simple off-the-shelf wavelength detector could report the same. There is no evidence that the photo device has an inner experience. You, however, can also report, "I have an inner, subjective awareness of green. I don't merely register the information that the apple is green; I *experience* it." Whatever that conscious feeling may be, that experiential component to green, it must be something that can in principle cause a verbal report. Of course, most subjective experiences are not verbally reported. It would be incorrect to equate awareness with verbal report. Nonetheless, awareness can in principle be verbally reported.

Some parts of consciousness, some things of which we are aware, are extremely hard to put into words. Try explaining colors to a congenitally blind person. (I actually tried this when I was about fourteen and lacked social tact. The conversation went in circles until I realized he did not have the concepts even to engage in the conversation, and I gave up.) However, as limited as human language is at information transfer, and as indescribable as some conscious experiences seem to be, we can nonetheless report that we have them. Consciousness can affect speech. It is tautologically true that all aspects of consciousness that we admit to having, that we report having, that we tell ourselves that we have, that philosophers and scientists write about having, that poets wax poetic about, can have some impact on language.

Speech is controlled by muscles, which are controlled by motorneurons, which are controlled by networks in the brain, which operate by computation and transmission of information. When you report that you have a subjective experience of greenness, information to that effect must have been present somewhere in the brain, passed to your speech circuitry, and translated into words. The brain contains information about awareness, encoded in the form of neural signals, or else we would be unable to report that we have it.

Even this preliminary realization, as obvious as it may seem, has a certain argumentative power. It rules out an entire class of theory. In my conversations with colleagues I often encounter a notion, sometimes implicitly assumed, sometimes explicitly articulated, that might be called the "emergent consciousness" concept. To summarize this type of view with extreme brevity: awareness is an aura or feeling that emerges from information-processing in the brain. When neurons in the brain are active in a certain pattern, the pattern generates or emits or allows for the feeling of awareness, a bit like heat emanating from electrical wires. Awareness is simply what it feels like to process information.

The difficulty with these common views is not so much in what they suggest as in what they leave out. These views acknowledge the presence of Arrow A (information leads to awareness), but they leave out any Arrow B. Awareness, having been generated by information, and being a feeling or an aura, an intangible experience, is unable to apply mechanical forces to alter a physical system and thus has no means to be turned back into information encoded in the brain. As a result, there is no mechanism for us to say that we have that awareness.

Strictly speaking, I am not arguing against the concept of an emergent awareness. It is acceptable for awareness to emerge from a physical process. But it must do more than emerge. Whatever emerges, it must also be able to impact the physical processes in the brain.

All theories of awareness that are unidirectional, that have an Arrow A but no Arrow B, are logically impossible. All workable theories of awareness must accommodate both an Arrow A and an Arrow B. Awareness must be able to act on the brain, to supply the brain with specific, reportable information about itself, or else we would be unable to say that we have it.

The Decision on Which the Report Is Based

Now let's take a second step into the brain, from the ability to report awareness to the ability to decide that we have awareness. If we can say that we have it, then prior to speech some processing system in the brain must have decided on the presence of awareness. Something must have supplied nonverbal information to the speech machinery to the effect that awareness is present, or else that circuitry would not be able to construct the verbal report.

All studies of awareness, whether philosophical pondering, introspection, or formal experiment, depend on a decision-making paradigm. A person decides, "Is awareness of X present?"

"Do I have a subjective experience of the greenness of the grass?"

"Do I have a subjective experience of the emotion of joy right now?"

"Do I merely register, in the sense of having access to the information, that the air I am breathing is cold, or do I actually have an experience of its coldness in my throat?"

"Do I have a subjective awareness of myself?"

All of these introspective queries are examples of decisions that can be made about the presence of awareness.

Here I would like to clarify exactly what I mean by a decision about the presence of awareness. Suppose that you are seated in front of a computer screen participating in an experiment. Images are flashed on the screen, one after the next, and your task is to indicate the color of each image. If it is red, you press one button. If it is green, you press a different button. The information that you are conveying by button press, the information that is the subject of your decision, concerns color, not awareness. You are probably also aware of the colors, at least at first. But after a few thousand trials you may go on autopilot, pressing, responding, doing quite well, while your conscious mind is elsewhere. In my experience, it is actually easier to perform a task like this when awareness has partially or even entirely left it.

If the images are flashed very briefly or are very dim, you may deny that anything was presented. But if forced to guess the color, you will probably be able to guess above chance. In that case, information about the image is present in your brain and can even result in a verbal report or a button press, while at the same time you are unable to detect a conscious experience attached to the color.

Merely being able to report that a visual stimulus is present, is of a certain color, has a certain shape, or is moving in a certain way is not the same as detecting the presence of awareness. A relatively simple machine that shows no evidence of awareness can be designed to detect low-level features, yet we humans can also detect and report on the presence of an inner experience.

Now imagine that the task is changed. The same type of image is flashed on the screen, but your job is to report whether you have a subjective experience of the image. You must introspect and decide if that special intangible stuff, awareness, is attached to the image. If yes, you press the response key. If not, naturally you skip the key press. Now the determination is not the presence of red or green, but the presence of awareness. If the images are presented slowly and clearly, and you are not overtaxed with thousands of trials, you will probably decide that awareness is present with each image. If the images are flashed too quickly or too dimly, or if you are distracted from the task, you may fail to detect any awareness, any inner experience, attached to the images.

The purpose of these elaborate examples is to isolate one specific type of decision. The brain can certainly decide whether something is green or red, big or small, important or unimportant, dangerous or safe, complicated or simple. But we can also decide that we have, within us, conscious experience of those things. Whatever the specific property of awareness may be, it is something that a brain can detect. We can decide that we have it.

Much has been learned recently about the neuronal basis of decision-making, especially in the relatively simple case of visual motion.[4,5] Suppose that you are looking at a blurry or flickering image and are asked to decide its direction of motion. It can drift either to the left or the right, but because of the noisy quality of the image, you have trouble determining the direction. By making the task difficult in this way, neuroscientists can slow down the decision process, thereby making it easier to study.

This decision process appears to work as follows. First, the machinery in the visual system constructs signals that represent the motion of the image. Because the visual image is noisy, it may result in conflicting signals indicating motion in a variety of directions. Second, those signals are received elsewhere in the brain by decision integrators. The decision integrators determine which motion signal is consistent enough or strong enough to cross a threshold. Once the threshold is crossed, a response is triggered. In this way, the system decides which direction the image is likely to be moving.

Strictly speaking, the system is not deciding whether the visual image is moving to the right or left. It is deciding between two information streams in the brain: is the left or right motion signal stronger? The decision can even be manipulated by inserting a fine electrode into the brain, into a particular part of the visual system, passing a very small electrical current and thereby boosting one or another of the motion signals.[6]

Since neuroscientists have some notion of the brain's machinery for decision-making, what can be inferred about awareness? As noted above, you can decide whether you have, inside of you, an awareness of something. Therefore awareness—or at least whatever it is you are deciding you have when you say you have awareness—can be fed into a decision integrator. We can make the task even more comparable to the visual-motion task. By making the images extremely brief or dim, we can make the task difficult. You may struggle for a moment, trying to decide whether any awareness of a stimulus is present. The decision machinery is engaged. This insight that conscious report depends on the machinery of decision-making has been pointed out before.[7,8]

A crucial property of decision-making is that not only is the decision itself a manipulation of data, but the decision machine depends on data as input. It does not take any other input. Feeding in some *res cogitans* will not work on this machine. Neither will Chi. You can't feed it ectoplasm. You can't feed it an intangible, ineffable, indescribable thing. You can't feed it an emergent property that transcends information. You can only feed it information.

In introspecting, in asking yourself whether you have an awareness of something, and in making the decision that you have it, what you are deciding on, what you are assessing, the actual *stuff* your decision engine is collecting, weighing, and concluding that you have, is information. Strictly speaking, the neuronal machinery is deciding that certain information is present in your brain at a signal strength above a threshold.

Now we are beginning to approach the counterintuitive concept that awareness—the mysterious stuff inside our heads, the private feeling we can talk about—might itself be information.

The Representation on Which the Decision Is Based

In the previous section I focused on the process of decision-making in the brain. I suggested that because we can *decide* that we have awareness, and because decisions require information, awareness might itself be information.

That reasoning may at first seem faulty. I will approach it here by first giving an obvious counterargument. Suppose that you are looking at a hunk of rock. You can decide that the rock is present and report that the rock is present, and yet the rock is not itself made of information. It's probably mostly silicate. (It could be argued that silicate, at the most esoteric level of quantum theory, is really just information; but I'll put that argument aside. The rock is not an informational representation in your brain to which you have cognitive access. It is an object in the real world.) This example seems to put the kybosh on the proposal that if you can decide it is there, then it must be information.

How can consciousness *be* information? Am I confusing information *about* a thing with the thing itself? Why can't consciousness be an aura, or a feeling, something that is not itself information but that can affect the brain, alter the signals, and thereby provide information about itself to the neuronal circuitry?

To get at the issue more clearly, consider the example of the rock a little more closely. Suppose you look and decide that a rock is indeed present in front of you. You can describe some of the properties of the rock. It's large, it's sparkling, it's white and gray, it's shaped like a lopsided triangle. Yet strictly speaking you are not deciding and reporting on the rock itself. You are deciding and reporting on the information constructed in your visual system.

To demonstrate the point, suppose you experience a visual illusion. A discrepancy is introduced between the real object and the visual representation of the object inside the brain. You look at a rock with illusory properties and are asked to report what is there. What do you report? Obviously, you report the informational representation, not the real thing. Due to a trick of perspective, you might decide it is triangular when it is actually square. You might decide it is smaller than your hand when it is actually larger than your whole body but much farther away than you think. Your decision machinery does not have direct access to the real object, only to the information about the object that is encoded in the visual system.

The issue runs deeper than occasional illusions in which a representation in the brain is incorrect. A perceptual representation is *always* inaccurate because it is a simplification. Let me remind you of an example from the previous chapter, the case of color and, in particular, the color white. Actual white light contains a mixture of all colors. We know it from experiment. But the model of white light constructed in the brain does not contain that information. White is not represented in the brain as a mixture of colors but as luminance that lacks all color. A fundamental gap exists between the physical thing being represented (a mixture of electromagnetic wavelengths) and the simplified representation of it in the brain (luminance without color). The brain's representation describes something in violation of physics. It took Newton[9] to discover the discrepancy.

(Newton's publication on color in 1671[9] was derided at the time, causing him much frustration. The philosophers and scientists of the Royal Society of London had trouble escaping their intuitive beliefs. They could not accept a mixture of colors as the basis for perceptual white. The difference between the real thing and the brain's internal representation was too great for them to grasp. For an account of this and other episodes in Newton's life, see the biography by Villamil.[10])

In the case of white light, we can distinguish between four items.

Item I is a real physical thing; a broad spectrum of wavelengths.

Item II is a representation in the brain's visual circuitry, information that stands for, but in many ways depicts something different from, the physical thing. The information depicts a simplified version, minus the physical details that are unimportant for one's own survival, and with no adherence to the laws of physics. What is depicted is in fact physically impossible. To be precise, we can distinguish two parts to Item II, let's say IIa and IIb. *Item IIa* is the information itself, which does exist and is instantiated in specialized circuitry of the visual system. *Item IIb* is the impossible entity depicted by that information—brightness without color.

Item III is the cognitive access to that representation, the decision-making process that allows the brain to scan the visual representation and abstract properties such as that a white surface is present or has a certain saturation or is located here or there in the environment.

Item IV is the verbal report.

In the case of looking at a rock, we have again *I,* a real physical thing; *II,* a representation in the brain that is a schematized, informational proxy for the real thing; *III,* a cognitive access to that representation; and *IV,* a verbal ability to report.

The division into four separate items is of course an egregious simplification of what is more like a continuous process, but the simplification helps to get at a deeper insight.

Consider the case of awareness. Suppose that there is a real physical basis for awareness, a mysterious entity that is not itself composed of information. Its composition is totally unknown. It might be a process in the brain, an emergent pattern, an aura, a subjectivity that is shed by information, or something even more exotic. At the moment suppose we know nothing about it. Let us call this thing Item I. Suppose that Item I, whatever it is, leaves information about itself in the brain's circuitry. Let us call this informational representation Item II. Suppose the informational representation can be accessed by decision machinery (Item III). Having decided that awareness is present, the brain can then encode this information verbally, allowing it to say that it is aware (Item IV). Where in this sequence is awareness? Is it the original stuff, Item I, that is the ultimate basis for the report? Is it the representation of it in the brain, Item II, that is composed of information? Is it the cognitive process, Item III, of accessing that representation and summarizing its properties? Or is it the verbal report, Item IV? Of course, we can arbitrarily define the word *awareness*, assigning it to any of these items. But which item comes closest to the common intuitive understanding of awareness?

Consider Item I. If there is such an entity from which information about awareness is ultimately derived, a real thing on which our reports of awareness are based, and if we could find out what that thing is, we might be surprised by its properties. It might be different from the information that we report on awareness. It might be something quite simple, mechanical, bizarre, or in some other way inconsistent with our intuitions about awareness. We might be baffled by the reality of Item I. We might be outraged by the identification, just as Newton's contemporaries were outraged when told that the physical reality of white light is a mixture of all colors. There is no reason to suppose that we would recognize Item I as awareness.

The thing to which the brain has cognitive access, and therefore the thing we describe when we report on awareness, is not Item I but rather the brain's informational depiction of it, Item II. The properties that we attribute to awareness are properties depicted in Item II.

The Real Item on Which the Representation Is Based

One does not need to look far for the Item I, the real item on which the report of awareness is based. Like seeing a rock and then investigating and finding out that what you see is not merely an illusion, that there is indeed a physical object in front of you, so too we can find that awareness is not merely an illusion with no basis but that it has a real, physical item on which the information is based.

Consider again the case of white light. Most of the time that people report the experience of white it is because a broadband mixture of wavelengths is available to the eyes. The match, incidence by incidence, is close. It is not exact because a perceptual model is not perfectly accurate. Sometimes people report seeing white in the absence of the expected physical stimulus. Sometimes the broadband stimulus is present and people report a different color. Visual illusions abound. But by and large, almost all the time, that physical stimulus causes perceptual white. The two are correlated.

Following the same logic, we should look for a physical, objectively measurable item that is almost always present when people report the presence of awareness. There is such an item, a physiological process in the brain, the process of attention. Almost uniformly, when you attend to an item, you report being aware of it.[11–14] The match, however, is not perfect. There are instances when it is possible to attend to something by all objective measures, meaning that your brain can selectively process it and react to it, and yet at the same time you report that you have no awareness of it.[11,12,15–17] These effects can occur in some cases of brain damage but can also be induced in normal healthy volunteers. Awareness and attention are therefore not the same, given that they can be separated. But they are typically associated. When the physical, measurable process of attention engages in the brain, when attention is directed at thing X, people almost always report the presence of awareness of thing X. For this reason, I argue that attention is Item I, the real physical item, a physical process, and awareness is Item II, the informational representation of it.

Attention, physiological attention as it is understood by neuroscientists, is a procedure. It is a competition between signals in the brain. It occurs because of the specific way that neurons interact with each other. One set of signals, carried by one set of neurons, rises in strength and suppresses other, competing signals carried by other neurons. For example, the visual system builds informational models of the objects in a scene. If you are looking at a cluttered scene, which informational model in your brain will win the competition of the moment, rise in signal strength, suppress other models, and dominate the brain's computations? This competition among signals—the process by which one signal wins and dominates for a moment, then sinks down as another signal dominates—is attention. Attention may be complicated, but it is not mysterious. It is physically understandable. It could be built into a circuit.

The correspondence between awareness and attention is close. In the previous chapter I outlined a list of similarities, and in later chapters I will discuss the relationship in greater detail. The two are so similar that it is tempting to think they might be the same thing with no distinction at all. But there is a fundamental difference. Attention, the competition among signals and the enhancement of signals in the brain, is a mechanistic process. It is not explicit knowledge. Awareness, in contrast, is accessible as explicit knowledge. The brain *does* attention but *knows* awareness.

The relationship between attention and awareness is therefore exactly the relationship between Item I and Item II, between a real thing and a representation of it in the brain that is cognitively accessible. Awareness, in this view, is a description, a useful if physically inaccurate sketch of what it means for the brain to focus its attention.

I imagine that most people will balk at the idea that awareness is based on the physical reality of a complicated, mechanistic, data-handling procedure in the brain. The one seems so ethereal and personal, the other so concrete and mundane. Likewise, Newton's contemporaries saw white light as ethereal, spiritual, deistic, and holy, and they saw a mixture of the colors, mashed together into one beam, as something dirty, mechanistic, reductionist, and simply impossible to imagine as the basis for white. But it is. When shown that physical item, people almost always generate the construct of white in their heads. Similarly, given the physical process of attention directed at thing X, the brain almost always constructs the reportable knowledge that it has an ethereal, subjective awareness focused on thing X.

The key to understanding the attention schema theory is to understand the distinction between the Item I being represented and the Item II that represents it. When we introspect, when we decide what is inside of us, the machinery of decision-making does not have direct access to Item I, the process of attention, because Item I is not itself accessible information. It is procedural. It is something the brain does, not something the brain knows. Instead, the cognitive machinery has access to Item II, and so when we decide what, exactly, we have inside of us, we arrive at the properties described by Item II. We report an experience, a feeling, an aura, something ethereal, something incorporeal, because that is the brain's schematized way to depict attention.

4

Being Aware versus Knowing that You Are Aware

In the previous chapter I suggested that awareness is information encoded in the brain. But am I mistaking awareness itself for the abstract knowledge that we have it? This chapter considers the distinction between *being* aware of something and *knowing* that you are aware of it.

The knowledge that you are conscious is an example of metacognition, or higher-order thought[1-3]—so-called thinking about thinking. I do not wish to give the incorrect impression that the attention schema theory is a metacognition theory of consciousness. In the present theory, behind the metacognition, behind the higher-order thought, behind the decision that you are conscious lies the attention schema.

In 1996, the philosopher Block[4] proposed that we have two kinds of consciousness. Intuitively we feel that we have a raw inner experience of colors, sounds, emotions, and other events (phenomenal consciousness); we also have a more abstract, cognitive ability to think about and report on those experiences (access consciousness). Does the attention schema theory equate consciousness with higher-order thought, akin to Block's access consciousness, or does it equate consciousness with something more raw and perceptual, akin to Block's phenomenal consciousness?

The attention schema theory arguably encompasses both. In the previous chapter I outlined a simplified way to divide the brain's processing of consciousness into Items I through IV. Here I suggest that Items I and II can be thought of as more like Block's phenomenal consciousness. They encompass the raw material (Item I) from which information about awareness is derived and a rich informational depiction of it (Item II). Items III and IV correspond more to Block's access consciousness. They encompass the cognitive capacity (Item III) to access that information set and extract summary information and the ability to formulate a verbal report (Item IV).

Suppose that you are looking at a living room. Your visual system contains information about the visual scene. Other processes in your brain are able to abstract from that data set. For example, if you are asked, "Which is taller: the lamp or the piano?" some set of cognitive processes in your brain can tap the trove of visuospatial information and compute that the lamp is taller, a simple relational proposition abstracted from the data set. Similarly, you may compute that the couch is to the left of the chair, another relational proposition abstracted from the data set. These verbalized reports represent a tiny fraction of the information present in the visual data set. It is no use trying to verbalize all the information in the data set. It can't be done. The data set is so rich and so analog in nature that it is not an easy fit to the constraints of language.

Awareness, in the present proposal, works something like the processing of a visual scene. The brain constructs a data set that paints a rich picture of your own attention directed at something, the spatial and temporal dynamics of your attention, the implications, the likely effects of it on behavior. The data set is so rich and complex that it is largely unverbalizable. This data set is comparable to Block's phenomenal consciousness. Other processes in the brain, cognitive processes, are able to access and abstract from that information set. For example, you might decide and report that you are aware of X, and that you are more aware of X than of Y. These decisions and summary statements are reminiscent of Block's access consciousness. They are cognition about consciousness. In this way, one could think of the present theory as encompassing both phenomenal consciousness and access consciousness.

I do not mean to put too much emphasis on a simple, rigid dichotomy between phenomenal consciousness and access consciousness. I am certain the reality is more complex than a dichotomy; in all likelihood, consciousness, like visual processing, cannot be accurately broken into a dichotomy. Perhaps a continuum of processing exists from a more raw informational model, through many degrees of abstraction, to the highest levels of cognitive operation such as formulating an explicit verbal report.

As an example of the mixing of levels in consciousness, suppose again that you are looking at a green apple. Your cognitive machinery can decide and report that you are aware of green. But you can also be aware of the deciding and aware of the reporting. The awareness feature can be applied to many of the intervening steps. It is not limited to the input end. The distinction between phenomenal consciousness on the one hand and the abstract knowledge that you are conscious on the other hand becomes rather fuzzy, since you can apply the one to the other. You can have phenomenal consciousness of your access consciousness. The neat divisions break down, and the dichotomy ceases to have much meaning.

If the dichotomy is iffy, then why bring up this concept of phenomenal consciousness and access consciousness? My point here is that, by suggesting that consciousness is information, I am not limiting the theory to cognition, abstraction, higher-order thought, simple verbalizable propositions, or access consciousness. The hypothesized attention schema, like a sensory representation, is a rich and constantly updated information set that can itself be accessed by cognitive processes. Because the attention schema is proposed to be similar to a sensory representation—because the brain uses the attention schema as a model for a physically real entity, just as it uses a sensory representation as a model for a physically real entity—the brain should have no basis for assigning the attention schema any less reality. In this theory, just as the brain takes the visual descriptions in visual circuitry as real things in a real world, so too the brain takes awareness, its representation of attention, as a real essence inside the body.

The attention schema theory could be said to lie half-way between two common views. In his groundbreaking book in 1991,[5] Dennett explored a cognitive approach to consciousness, suggesting that the concept of qualia, of the inner, private experiences, is incoherent and thus we cannot truly have them. Others, such as Searle,[6] suggested that the inner, subjective state exists by definition and is immune to attempts to explain it away. The present view lies somewhere in between; or perhaps, in the present view, the distinction between Dennett and Searle becomes moot. In the attention schema theory, the brain contains a representation, a rich informational description. The thing depicted in such nuance is experienceness. Is it real? Is it not? Does it matter? If it is depicted then doesn't it have a type of simulated reality?

If awareness is Item IIb, the impossible, private, lovely thing that is depicted by the information of Item IIa, then whether awareness exists or not becomes philosophically murky. It is described by the brain, not produced by the brain. It exists only as a simulation. Yet because the item that is described is so gauzy, so ethereal, and so much like a simulation one must ask: if it is simulated, and if it is supposed to be a thing like a simulation, then does it not actually exist?

My point here is that it is possible to be mechanistic and philosophical at the same time. The attention schema theory provides a specific, mechanistic account of awareness, of its brain basis, what it is made out of and how we are able to report it. The theory depends on nothing beyond the nuts and bolts of neurons transmitting and computing information. Yet we still have room for some philosophical nuance.

I am reminded of Magritte's famous painting, *The Treachery of Images*. He painted a pipe with impressive realism and beneath it painted the words, "Ceci n'est pas une pipe." This is not a pipe. Technically, it is a representation of a pipe, not a pipe itself. Magritte said, "The famous pipe. How people reproached me for it!"[7] If people have trouble agreeing on the existential reality of a pipe beautifully rendered in a painting, think how much harder it is to agree on the existential reality of a beautiful awareness rendered or described by information in the brain. It is real. It isn't real. The attention schema theory does not even seek to answer the question of its existential reality but instead tries to describe what is constructed by the brain. One could think of awareness as information. One could also think of it as the lovely ghost described by that information.

5

The Attention Schema

The heart of the theory is that awareness is a schematized, descriptive model of attention. The model is not perfectly accurate, but it is good enough to be useful. It is a rich information set, as rich as a sensory representation. It can be bound to a representation of an object as though it were another sensory attribute like color or motion. That added information can inform higher-order, cognitive processes, thereby allowing us to decide and conclude and believe and report that we are aware of something. The purpose of the present chapter is to explore further what that model might be like and what its components might be.

Generally, when the brain constructs an informational representation of something, the adaptive advantage is obvious. The brain constructs informational models of entities in the real world. Those models can be manipulated or consulted in order to plan actions or make predictions. In this sense one's cognitive processes are like generals in a war room pushing models of soldiers and tanks around a map. Obviously, a green plastic army man is different from an actual human soldier; but for the purpose of planning strategy, it can do very well. Similarly, the purpose of a model in the brain is to be useful in interacting with the world, not to be accurate.

Here I would like to clarify what I mean by "model" since the word is used in different ways in different scientific subdisciplines.

I mean something close to the colloquial term. I mean something reduced, simplified, and convenient, that represents something else more complicated, like a model airplane represents a real airplane, or a plastic soldier represents a real one. A model in the brain, in this use of the word, is an information set that is constructed and constantly updated by neuronal machinery and that represents something useful to monitor and predict. A similar use of the word can be found in Johnson-Laird's classic book on metal models.[1]

If awareness is information, if it is a rich informational model akin to a sensory model, then what is its counterpart in the real world? What is it a model of? The heart of the theory is that awareness is a model of attention. The purpose of this chapter is to provide a brief overview of attention, to discuss the possible adaptive advantages of modeling it, and to begin to outline some of the properties that a model of it might contain.

What Is Attention and Why Is It Useful to Model?

As I noted before, the word *attention* has many meanings, especially in colloquial English. I use the word in a neuroscientific sense. I am referring to a mechanistic process in the brain. Attention can be understood at least partly through a theoretical framework called biased competition.[2-4] The biased-competition framework was developed by studying the case of visual attention. Normally, many visual stimuli are in front of us at the same time, and therefore the brain constructs many representations. These representations of stimuli compete with each other. They inhibit each other. As one representation rises up in strength and wins the competition, it suppresses other representations.

This competition can be influenced by a variety of signals. One type of signal is called bottom-up. A bottom-up signal might be, for example, the brightness or the sudden onset of a stimulus, which can cause the representation of that stimulus in the brain to gain signal strength and win the competition. A second type of signal is called top-down. An example of a top-down signal is a choice to look at a region of space, for example, choosing to look on your bedside table to find your glasses. Another example of a top-down signal is a choice to look through a crowd specifically for a man in a red hat.

The combination of top-down and bottom-up signals will bias the competition in favor of one or another stimulus representation. Once a sensory representation has won the competition and its signal strength is boosted, that representation is much more likely to drive the behavior of the animal. It is shouting louder than other signals. Its greater strength allows it to influence other circuitry in the brain. This self-organizing process is constantly shifting as one or another representation temporarily wins the competition.

In essence, attention is a process by which a brain seizes on a signal, focuses its intelligent computation on that signal, processes the signal in a deep manner, has its cognitive machinery driven by that signal, and tends to control behavior on the basis of that signal. The target of attention need not be a visual stimulus. Indeed, it need not even be any kind of sensory stimulus. It is possible to attend to an idea, a movement, an emotion, a belief, a memory, a smell, a taste, a sound, a sight, or an object that combines all of those properties. Attention is a general way to handle data and can apply to a range of information domains. It is an enhancement operation and a selection operation performed on signals in the brain.

Attention, especially visual attention, has been heavily studied, and a great deal has been written about it. I would like to focus on one aspect of attention that is not usually considered: its usefulness in predicting behavior. If you could know one thing about an animal to best predict its behavior, I suggest that attentional state would be the wisest choice. If you could know what the animal is attending to, how much of its attention is allocated to the item, and what the consequences of attention are, then you would gain considerable ability to predict the animal's behavior. The reason is simply that attended items drive more of the processing in the brain than unattended items and thus tend to drive the animal's behavior.

For example, if I am an antelope in the veldt and see a lion, it is useful for me to know whether that lion's attention is focused on me or on something else. It is useful for me to understand the basic dynamics of attention.

If I am a monkey with a bad wound on my leg and a subordinate monkey comes near, it is useful for me to know if my wound is in the purview of the other monkey's attention. If so, then I might expect a challenge to my dominant position. If not, then I can bluff my way through the interaction.

If I am single at a party and looking for somebody to date, it may be useful for me to know whether this or that woman's attention is slyly directed at me.

If I am fighting for my life with a home invader, it is extremely useful for me to know whether the bad guy's attention has shifted to the knife that happens to be lying in the kitchen sink. It will determine my strategy in the fight.

Suppose I am at a party. If I am on a diet, and I find myself paying close attention to a plate of colorful sugar-coated doughnuts that somebody has left on the table, if I find that I can't get them out of my mind, if I find they are capturing my attention, then I can make a good prediction about my own likely short-term behavior. I might decide to move away from that part of the room or move to a different room altogether to get them out of my sight, out of my mind—out of my attention.

The above examples are rather specialized. I suggest that, in general, to predict and therefore effectively interact with an intelligent brain-controlled agent, it is useful to construct and constantly update a model of the shifting state of that agent's attention. Just as much, in planning your own behavior, it is critical to have a good predictive model of your own likely actions; therefore, it is useful to construct a model that represents your own attention.

In the attention schema theory, awareness serves this function. It is a vast, rich, constantly updated informational model whose purpose is to usefully describe the constantly changing state of attention.

Comparison of the Attention Schema to the Body Schema

A schema is a complex information structure that is used to represent something. One of the first schemas to be extensively studied in psychology and neuroscience was the body schema, first proposed by Head and Holmes in 1911.[5] To clarify exactly what I mean by a schema and how a schema can be useful to the brain, I will explain some of the basics of the body schema, a topic on which I've worked and published over many years.[6] The body schema and the attention schema may share more than a formal similarity. They may partially overlap.

The body schema is an internal model—an organized set of information that represents the shape, structure, and movement of the body, that distinguishes between objects belonging to the body and objects that are foreign.

It is easy to confuse the body schema with low-level sensing. The body is filled with mechanical sensors that indicate the angles of joints and positions of limbs. That sensory information must be put together somehow in the brain. The representation of the body, however, is more complex than a mere registry of joint angles. It incorporates information from many sources. For example, you can learn about the position of your arm by looking at it. You can learn about the position of your legs by extrapolating from the movement commands that you recently sent to them. You can deduce something about the state of your body by using basic knowledge about its jointed structure. Your brain pulls together a diversity of information and uses it to build an elaborate, inner model of your physical self, of its current state and its possible future states. That model is the body schema. Figure 5.1 diagrams this concept of many sources of information converging on a central body schema.

One of the most charming demonstrations of the body schema is the so-called Pinocchio illusion.[7] A person closes his eyes and touches his nose with the tip of his index finger. While the person holds that pose, the experimenter uses a vibrator to vibrate a tendon in the arm.

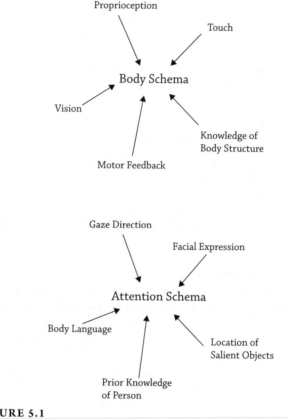

FIGURE 5.1

Comparison of the body schema and the attention schema.

The tendon vibration produces a false signal that the elbow joint is rotating and therefore that the arm is extending. Now the person's body schema is faced with incompatible information. He can feel the tip of his finger against the tip of his nose. Yet if his elbow is extending, then his hand must be moving away from his face. The result? "Doctor, my nose is growing! I feel like Pinocchio!" The body schema recalibrates its representation of the size and shape of the relevant body part. The illusion does not work the same way for everybody. The body schemas of different people seem to adjust different parts of the representation. For some people the index finger feels longer, and for some people the effect of the tendon vibration is suppressed and the arm feels stationary. All of these outcomes are the result of the brain doing the best it can to compute the most accurate configuration of the body, the most accurate body schema, while juggling conflicting information.

Another now-classic demonstration of the body schema is the rubber hand illusion.[8] A person sits at a table with her left hand in her lap. Her right hand is resting on the table. The person cannot see her right hand—it's covered by cardboard—but she can see a fake, rubber hand lying on the table, arranged plausibly, sometimes sticking out of a sleeve, so that it could stand in for her own right hand. She knows cognitively that it is fake. Nobody is trying to fool her. And indeed, she has no sense whatsoever that this lifeless rubber hand belongs to her. Now the experimenter picks up a small paintbrush and begins to stroke the rubber hand from the wrist to the knuckles, from the knuckles to the tip of the index finger, and back. At the same time, out of view, the experimenter strokes the subject's real hand in precisely the same way. Stroke for stroke, the subject of the experiment feels a paint brush moving across her own hand and sees a paint brush moving across the fake hand. After a few minutes, an uncanny illusion develops. The rubber hand begins to feel like the subject's own. This illusion is almost impossible to describe unless you experience it yourself. You know, intellectually, that the rubber hand is rubber. It isn't yours. And yet a powerful sense comes over you that it *is* yours. It is a part of your body. A threat to it is a threat to you. This illusion is another example of the body schema reconciling conflicting information, in this case the sight of the brush on the rubber hand and the feel of the brush on your own hand.

The rubber hand illusion has now been studied in many variants. At one point my own lab studied a set of neurons in the brain that may supply part of the machinery behind the rubber hand illusion.[9,10] Others have extended the rubber hand illusion to create a false sense of ownership over an arm, a torso, or an entire manikin body.[11]

The body schema is thought to be useful in a variety of ways. For example, in 1911, Head and Holmes[5] noted that women who wore large hats with protruding feathers could get into coaches and walk through doorways without breaking their feathers. The behavior suggested that the feathered hat had been incorporated into the body schema. Similar examples abound. When driving, we seem to "sense" the boundaries of the car, keeping a safe distance from obstacles. Examples of this type suggest that the body schema can help to maintain a margin of safety around the various parts and extensions of the body.

This classic view, that the body schema is used to maintain a margin of safety around the body, is in some ways naïve. It is too narrow a window on the body schema. We now know from control theory that almost any movement can be controlled better and more flexibly if the control system can tap into a body schema. One does not need to resort to the exotic example of feathered hats. Just reaching for a coffee cup will do as well.

The body schema does not merely monitor the state of the body. The word *monitoring* implies too trivial a process. A model of a complex system, such as a computer model of the weather, can imitate the dynamics and allow for predictions; a mere monitoring process cannot. In movement control, when trying to control an arm, for example, a distinction can be made between feedback about the state of the arm (monitoring or tracking the arm) and constructing an internal model of the arm (computing a simulation of the arm). The usefulness of an internal model that can predict movement at least a few seconds into the future is now generally understood.[12,13]

Movement control is not the only possible use for a body schema. It also may play a role in understanding the bodies of other people. For example, if you view a picture of someone else's hand and are asked to decide if it is a left hand or a right hand, the easiest approach, and the approach that most people evidently take, is to imagine rotating your own right or left hand until it matches the configuration in the picture.[14,15] The typical approach, therefore, is to use your own hand schema to think about or judge someone else's hands. When people perform this task, regions of the brain that are believed to be involved in the body schema become active.[16]

When my own lab studied the body schema, we encountered the following spooky experience. Take a person, tuck his arms in his shirt, and place false arms on him. Switch the arms, such that the left arm is on the right and vice versa. Somebody else looking at that person may not be able to spot the switch immediately. But the realization that *something* is wrong will jump out. Alternatively, watch a double-jointed person bend her elbow backward. The thought of it isn't so bad, but to actually see it gives you the heebie jeebies. These colorful examples illustrate a property of the body schema: we seem to use our model of a body, of the normal physical structure and movement of the human body, to evaluate the state of other people's bodies. In this sense, the body schema can act like a general perceptual engine. It can be used to model oneself or to model the bodies of others.

In the present theory, the attention schema is similar to the body schema. Rather than representing one's physical body, it models a different aspect of oneself, also a complex dynamical system, the process of attention—the process by which some signals in the brain become enhanced at the expense of others. It is a predictive model of attention, its dynamics, its essential meaning, its potential impact on behavior, what it can and can't do, what affects it, and how. It is a simulation. The quirky way that attention shifts from place to place, from item to item, its fluctuating intensity, its spatial and temporal dynamics—all of these aspects are incorporated into the model.

Like the body schema, the proposed attention schema integrates many sources of information. If you are observing Susan, to construct a model of her attention might require information about where she is looking, her facial expression, her body language, her speech, the objects around her at the moment, and your prior knowledge about her. These many sources of information converge and constrain your model of her attention. Whatever machinery computes the attention schema must integrate multiple cues. This comparison between the body schema and the attention schema is diagrammed in Figure 5.1.

Several other researchers have suggested that awareness might be an internal model of attention.[17,18] These previous accounts are based on robotics and optimal-control theory. In these accounts, we use awareness as a guide signal to control our own attention. In the same way, we use an internal model of the arm to help control the actual arm. I am obviously a fan of this prior research because of its similarity to my own proposal. But I think the previous suggestions are too limited. They do not capture the complexity or broad usefulness of a model of attention.

The attention schema theory goes beyond robotics, beyond control theory, beyond the specific goal of regulating this or that internal parameter. I am suggesting that the attention schema has a more general role in understanding, predicting, and guiding behavior. It is a sophisticated model of one of the most fundamental aspects of brain function. It can be used to understand one's own and other people's mind states, to understand the dynamics of shifting attention and shifting thought, to understand and predict decisions, to understand and predict actions. It is the brain's working description of what it means for a brain to seize on information, focus on it, and deeply process it. The next two chapters describe more of the possible properties and details of the attention schema.

6

Illusions and Myths

The theory proposed in this book can be summarized in five words: awareness is an attention schema. A schema is an informational model, constantly recomputed, that represents something worth tracking and predicting. The proposed attention schema is a set of information, call it *A*, that represents attention. But the representation has its own idiosyncratic, even extravagant properties that distinguish it from the mechanistic and complicated item being represented. What is included in the information set *A*? This chapter explores how our intuitions, cultural myths, and illusions concerning awareness might reveal something about the content of the proposed attention schema.

Neuroscience has spent more than a century studying the information content of representations in the brain. These studied representations include, for example, visual, tactile, auditory, emotional, and entirely abstract representations in various parts of the brain. I could write a multi-volume textbook on the information contained in a visual representation and how that information is computed and transformed in successive stages in the brain. Awareness, however, is a different matter. The information content of awareness is not studied. The reason, of course, is that most scientists and most thinkers on the topic have never considered awareness to be composed of information. Awareness is assumed to be something else, something extra, something that emanates from information or that takes in information or that hitches a ride alongside information. That awareness might itself be descriptive information has generally not been considered.

Here I am suggesting that awareness is indeed a chunk of information constructed in the brain. To be clear, I am not talking about the information that we normally think of as being "in" consciousness. If I ask myself what information is in my consciousness at this particular moment, I might say visual information, sound information, information about myself, my body, my emotions, my thoughts, and so on. I am conscious of all of that content. But in addition to the informational content of consciousness, according to the theory, my brain also constructs a set of information, A, that allows me to conclude that I am aware of the content.

What is the information that defines awareness itself? What is in the information set A? An easy, initial approach to the question is to examine the reports that people typically make when talking about awareness. Our verbal descriptions of it and our cultural mythology about it presumably reflect the contents of that information set as abstracted, summarized, schematized, and slightly garbled through the cognitive machinery of introspection and linguistic embedding. The present chapter examines some of these commonly reported intuitions and myths and on that basis draws some tentative inferences about the informational content of A.

The Out-of-Body Illusion

Intuitively we experience awareness as a thing located inside us or emanating from us. Its location inside the body is so obvious that we don't normally think much about it. But the spatial structure of awareness becomes more obvious when something goes wrong and that spatial structure is disrupted in an illusion. In the out-of-body experience, awareness is mislocalized to a place outside the body.[1]

Out-of-body experiences are traditionally reported in states close to sleep or near death or under partial anesthesia. One difficulty with studying this type of experience is that the mental functions of the person are so impaired that it is difficult to accept the report. It is difficult to disentangle a genuine perceptual illusion from a garbled account or a confused memory. However, the out-of-body experience can be induced reliably in a laboratory by putting people in a highly controlled, virtual-reality environment and by manipulating visual feedback and somatosensory feedback.[2,3] People can be made to feel as though they are floating in empty space or even as though they were magically transported to a location inside of another body. The self feels as though it is somewhere other than inside one's proper body.

An out-of-body illusion can also be induced by applying electrical stimulation to a specific region of the cerebral cortex. In one experiment, the scientist Blanke and colleagues[4] electrically stimulated the cortical surface of a human subject whose brain was temporarily exposed during a medically required surgery. As is typical during such brain surgeries, the patient was under local anesthesia and was therefore awake and able to report experiences. Electrical stimulation was applied to the surface of the cortex on the right side of the brain in a specific region called the temporo-parietal junction (TPJ). The stimulation temporarily scrambled the natural signals in this brain area. As a result, an out-of-body experience was induced. The patient felt as though she were floating outside her own body. The stimulation evidently interfered with the machinery that normally assigns a location to one's own mind.

The out-of-body illusion highlights a specific property of awareness: awareness comes with a computed spatial arrangement. Evidently, machinery in the brain computes one's awareness and assigns it a perceived source inside one's body, and interference with the relevant circuitry results in an error in the computation. The out-of-body illusion therefore reveals something quite specific about the information set, A, that defines awareness. That information set must include spatial information. Awareness is computed to be a thing that exists roughly *here*, at this or that location. The location is not so precisely defined as a point in space. Instead it is vaguely inside the body, usually inside the head.

Blanke and colleagues[5] suggested that there is a primacy to constructing a body-centered understanding of oneself, a model of oneself as a physical being with a location and a specific spatial perspective on the external world. Constructing this physical understanding of the self is, in their view, important to the construction of consciousness. This view is certainly consistent with the attention schema theory. Awareness is a computed property, and at least one part of it is a computed spatial embodiment.

The Feeling of Being Stared At

When you have a face-to-face conversation with another person, so many perceptions and cognitive models are present regarding tone of voice, facial expression, gesture, and the semantic meaning of the other person's words that it is difficult to isolate the specific perceptual experience of the other person's awareness. Yet there is one circumstance in which extraneous perceptions are minimized and the perception of someone else's awareness is relatively isolated and thus more obvious. Most people are familiar with the feeling that someone is staring at them from behind.[6,7] Although some mystics may believe this to be an instance of the supernatural, perhaps a direct sensing of someone else's thoughts, the phenomenon seems instead to be more mundane. Context, expectation, and subtle sounds and shadows form the physical basis of it, as Titchner found in his experiments more than a hundred years ago.[7]

Because the feeling that someone is staring at you is so linked to the pseudoscientific fringe, it has unfortunately been largely ignored by scientists for a century. The phenomenon is actually quite interesting. Some set of conditions affects the relevant circuitry in the brain and triggers the construction of a model of awareness. In that model, a mind is located behind you and is aware of you. This model of a mind is a type of social perception and a particularly pure case of attributing awareness. Other aspects of social perception are stripped away. The model that you construct includes the property of awareness, a rough spatial source of the awareness behind you, and a target of the awareness on the back of your head. The model has a distinctive spatial structure: a source, a target, and a vector leading from the one to the other.

The illusion helps to demonstrate that when computing someone else's attentional state, we do not merely construct the abstract proposition "Person X is attending to thing Y." It is not solely higher-order cognition or higher-order thought. We construct a rich perception-like model that includes a spatial embodiment. Indeed, we may know cognitively, with our higher-order thought, that nobody else is present and yet still have that creepy impression.

The Extromission Myth of Vision

The extromission myth of vision is the myth that we see by means of some substance that emanates out of the eyes and touches objects. Gross[8] reviewed the history of this myth. It was seriously considered as a theory of vision, or at least one of several competing theories of vision, by the ancient Greek philosophers. It was refuted scientifically by the thirteenth-century Arabic scientist Alhazen, who developed an essentially modern understanding of optics. Yet, even though the myth was debunked scientifically, it remains embedded in human culture.

For example, almost all cultures include a belief in the evil eye.[9] The evil eye refers to a malign, invisible influence that emanates from certain people's eyes and is especially harmful to children. The evil eye is not an antiquated belief. It remains common among a range of modern cultures, including Indo-European and Semitic cultures. Amulets to ward off the evil eye are also common.

The psychologist Piaget noted that when school children are asked to explain vision, they often describe something emanating out of the eyes.[10] Building on that finding, in the 1990s Winer and Cottrell[11-13] found that extromission views are common among American elementary school children. About 57% of them expressed the view that vision involves a substance coming out of the eyes. Even more shocking, about 33% of college students chose the same description. These studies were conducted fifteen years ago, not during some distant benighted historical epoch. The subjects were modern students in American colleges. When the question was asked in a variety of ways to avoid misunderstanding, and when the students were asked to draw pictures and arrows to clarify their responses, the results were essentially the same. Even students who had recently been taught basic science or basic physiology often chose an extromission account over an intromission account. The widespread belief in extromission is all the more remarkable given that the correct account is conceptually easy to understand and is taught at all school grade levels. As expressed by Winer and colleagues, "the source and apparent strength of extromission beliefs in children and adults is somewhat of a mystery."[13]

I suggest a simple explanation to the mystery. The myth of extromission is an abstract version, a cognitive summary, of an underlying model that the brain constructs to represent visual attention. The model is not physically accurate, but since it is built into us it is unavoidable. It is like the universal perception that white is pure and lacking any color, a physically incoherent mistake based on the model of white light constructed in the human visual system. No matter how well we understand the physical reality in a cognitive sense, we cannot eliminate a built-in perception. We can understand it to be scientifically wrong while accepting it to be perceptually true.

So far in this chapter I've briefly discussed the out-of-body experience, the feeling of being stared at, and now the extromission myth of vision. These strange but common experiences, I suggest, come about because our brains naturally depict attention, especially visual attention, as something that emanates from a source, travels through space, and arrives at a target. Though nonsensical from the point of view of physics, this simplified schema is actually a convenient way to keep track of who is attending to what. Again, the purpose of a perceptual model in the brain is not to be slavishly true to the physical reality in all its details but to be useful.

Mesmerism

The intuition that we can feel someone else's gaze on us or that some psychological force emanates from people and touches other people seems to have a hold on the human imagination. One of the more intriguing episodes in the history of science, or pseudoscience, is the story of mesmerism. In the 1770s, the physician Anton Mesmer claimed to have found a special, invisible force that emanates from or is influenced by animal tissue. He called it animal magnetism.[14]

At that time, Coulomb had recently discovered the mathematical laws that govern electrical forces. Magnetism was considered to be another fundamental force of nature, though Faraday had not yet formulated its fundamental equations. Galvani had recently used an electrical source to shock the severed legs of frogs, thereby causing the legs to kick.[15] Galvani's discovery was arguably the beginning of modern neurophysiology. It was a milestone in medical science. It also, incidentally, helped to set the stage for Mary Shelly's novel *Frankenstein*, published in 1818,[16] in which the famous monster, sewn together from miscellaneous parts of cadavers, was brought to life by electrical current. The idea that electricity, magnetism, and the secret energy of life were interrelated was in the cultural air.

In that climate, Mesmer began to experiment with passing iron bars over his hysterical and delusional patients, who often went into fits, spasms, and faints as a result.[17,18] He announced that he had discovered a new force of nature, animal magnetism, and continued to refine the "science" until he had a large and lucrative clientele. He eventually dispensed with iron bars and magnets and claimed that his hands were good enough conductors of animal magnetism for his medical purposes. People could palpably feel the energy coming from him. In his account, the force could pass through walls and closed doors.

In 1784, the king of France was so impressed by the popularity of the fad that he commissioned a scientific team to investigate it. (The team included Benjamin Franklin.) The report of the commission, which makes for rather fascinating reading, concluded that mesmerism seemed to be mainly imagination and under controlled tests its "energy" never did pass through a wall or a door and never did work on blindfolded people who were not informed that a source of magnetism was nearby. In short, it was largely fraud mixed up with a fascinating, poorly understood, but potent tendency toward suggestibility and mass human irrationality. The human mind seemed primed to believe in an invisible force that could emanate from one person and affect another.

The mysterious force, I suggest, is awareness. It originates in each person, can flow out of a person, and can touch another person. Of course I am not suggesting that any force actually emanates from one person to affect another. But I am suggesting that mesmerism depended on a basic property of human social perception. We are primed to perceive human awareness in this manner, as an energy-like plasma that can flow from person to person, because our perceptual machinery naturally constructs that type of model. Indeed, the belief is so natural that mesmerism continues to be popular today.[17]

The Myth of Psychokinesis

Almost everyone who casually thinks about consciousness assumes that consciousness can directly cause actions. Consciousness can move things. We consciously choose to move a hand, and lo, it moves. From that everyday notion, psychokinesis, the supposed ability to move things at a distance with thought, is merely an extrapolation. It may be pseudoscience, and it may be within the domain of charlatans and illusionists, but the belief is culturally widespread and historically old. It is shockingly easy to convince people that they are psychokinetic by rigging an experimental setup and tricking them with a few well-timed coincidences.[19,20]

An example from modern culture comes to mind. In a charming Super Bowl ad for Volkswagon, a little boy dressed as Darth Vader tries a mind trick on the family car. To his amazement, when he gestures and glares, the car turns on. He's psychokinetic! Either that or his sneaky father, watching from inside the house, has used the remote control. This vignette works on many levels, but one part of its appeal is that it connects to something we all understand. People have an intuitive grasp of psychokenesis. Children are especially gullible about the mind force and require some experience to learn that it is not so.

In common mythology, therefore, when you focus your awareness on something, you can move it. Awareness not only takes impressions from the physical world but it also pushes on the physical world.

My Head Hurts from Thinking Too Much

Consider a curious, common experience: someone who is thinking too hard might put a hand to his or her head and say, "My head hurts. It feels like it's going to explode!" I felt this way a few times while writing this book.

A favorite question of those who study consciousness could be put like this: why does information processing in the brain *feel* like anything at all? How come the information isn't simply manipulated, machine-like, without an inner feeling?

To me, this question conflates two issues. First, why do we have an inner experience at all? Second, why do we usually compare the inner experience to a kind of touch?

Most of this book is focused on the first question—why do we have an inner experience at all?—and I've suggested the attention schema theory as a possible answer. Here I would like to focus on the narrower, much less mysterious but nonetheless interesting second question: why do we compare awareness to a felt event?

We rarely say, "My awareness *looks* like it is inside my head," or, "My awareness *sounds* like it is inside me." An out-of-body experience never involves *tasting* your awareness to be in the upper corner of the room. In fact, such comments seem ridiculous because of their literal falsity. Instead, we feel. We *feel* awareness to be inside us. Awareness seems to be linked in a special way to the somatosensory domain. Somatosensory information may be a crucial part of the weave of information that composes A.

In previous sections of this chapter I discussed the spatial structure of awareness. We intuitively understand awareness to emanate from a location inside us. Part of constructing the feature of awareness is attributing it to a specific location inside the body. In this sense awareness is another example of a body sense such as touch. It is a representation of the workings of the inner environment. Like a sensory representation of a stomachache, or of joint rotation, or of a pressure headache behind the eyeballs, or of being cold or hot, one's own awareness is a representation of an event (physiological attention) that occurs inside the body. In this way awareness certainly resembles a feeling more than a sight or a sound. The culturally common analogy that we *feel* awareness inside us makes sense.

But the idea that we feel awareness may be more than an analogy. It may have a literal component. Drawing attention to your hand makes you feel your hand a little more vividly. Merely flashing a light near your hand will cause your brain to enhance the processing of touch on your palm.[21] Likewise, by localizing your awareness to the inside of your head, you may subtly, but literally, feel something touching or pressing inside your head. Awareness may come with rich informational associations to touch, temperature, pressure, perhaps even pain. All of these internal senses may be subtly primed and subtly activated along with the localization of awareness to the inside of the body.

The Physical Properties Attributed to Awareness

What do these culturally universal myths and illusions reveal about awareness?

In the present theory, awareness is information. It is an informational model in the human brain. The item described by that model is attention—the process by which a brain enhances signals. But the description is only a crude sketch and in many ways does not match attention. The model describes something remarkable, strange, physically impossible, and loosely based on the dynamics of attention.

Awareness, the model, lacks all the mechanistic details of neurons and competing signals in the brain. The physical nuts and bolts of attention are not present in the model. Why would an organism need to know those mechanistic details? Instead the essential dynamics of attention are duplicated in the model. According to the information set A, awareness is when an intelligence seizes on something. It is when a mind experiences something. It is a directing of mental effort onto something. An agent directs awareness at a target. The awareness itself has a physical structure. It has a location. It is a substance like ectoplasm that applies a subtle pressure or heat to the inside of the head, that emanates from the head, that flows through space, that can sometimes physically touch or push on things. Awareness is a fictionalized sketch of attention. It is an effective way to keep track of the essentials.

Let us use the term *substance A* to refer to the physically impossible entity that is described by the information set A. Substance A has a strong resemblance to *res cogitans*, the fluid substance of the soul that Descartes described. It is ectoplasm. It is spirit. It is the stuff that angels, ghosts, and gods are made of. It is the stuff that, in most cultures and most religions, is supposed to survive the death of the body.

I am not proposing that the brain contains spirit. I am proposing that the brain constructs an informational model and the information describes spirit more or less as people have intuitively understood it for millennia.

I noted in a previous chapter that, before Newton, people intuitively understood white to be "pure" or lacking all color. Most of us still tend to think of white in that fashion even though we know better intellectually. The reason for the universality and persistence of this belief is that the visual system naturally encodes it in that manner. The signal channel that represents luminance is at a high setting, and the signal channels that represent colors are set low. The brain constructs an informational model of a physically impossible pure, colorless luminance that we call white. In a similar way, in the present hypothesis, people intuitively understand consciousness to be spirit-like because the informational representation in the brain encodes it in that manner. In this view the spirit concept—the diaphanous invisible stuff that thinks and perceives and flows plasma-like through space and time, that can take impressions from the outside world, that can sometimes push on real objects, that normally inhabits the human body but can sometimes flow outside of it, and that therefore ought to be able to survive the death of the body—this myth so ubiquitous in human culture is not a mistaken belief, a naïve theory, or the result of superstitious ignorance, as many scientists would claim. It is instead a verbalization of a naturally occurring informational model in the human brain.

In this view, the mystery surrounding consciousness stems in part from a logical contradiction. Consciousness is composed of information that says, in effect, "This information is not information." In describing itself as something else, as a fluidic substance, as an experience, as sentience, it is declaring itself not to be information. It is self-contradictory information. It says, "I am not me," or, "P is not P." No wonder so much logical confusion ensues. On introspection, that is to say on scanning the relevant internal data, the brain finds no basis whatsoever for concluding that awareness is merely information because the information does not describe itself that way.

Most scientists who study consciousness tend to pick and choose among intuitions. The intuition that consciousness is a substance inside of me, or that it can flow outside of me, or that it can directly touch another person and alert him or her is dismissed as obviously scientifically impossible. That is magic. That is ghost material. Modern scientists are emancipated from ghost mythology. But the intuition that consciousness is subjective, private, an inner experience, a feeling, an intelligence that takes in information, is often accepted as a fundamental assumption, a mystery to be explained. I am suggesting here that all of these introspected attributes of consciousness, whether they seem reasonable or seem magical, are equally based on a cognitive access to and a summary of a deeper data set in the brain. The brain has constructed a model of something, a picture painted in the medium of information. The model is not terribly accurate. At least, the biophysics of neurons and signals are nowhere described in that model. But the model is nonetheless useful because it keeps track of the essential dynamics and the behavioral consequences of attention.

7

Social Attention

The theory that awareness is a model of attention has a certain advantage. The human brain is known to construct just such a model of attention. The machinery exists. The capability is there. It has been studied in the context of social thinking. Humans have the ability to construct a model of someone else's attentional state.[1-5]

Imagine that you are observing Bill. You see him look here and there. You see his facial expression and body language. You hear what he has to say. Obviously you can infer something about his attentional state. You can probably guess what he is attending to and even what he may attend to next. I am on safe ground with those assertions. But what kind of mental model have you constructed? When you reconstruct the state of his attention, where does that mental model stand on the scale from the perceptual to the cognitive? Does Bill's awareness have a quality of physical reality to you, a thing that exists inside Bill, or does it seem more like your own clever deduction, an abstract proposition in your own head? Is it better described as social perception or social cognition?

For many scientists, there is little difference between social perception and social cognition. The brain constructs many different models of other people's minds, and the models exist at different levels of abstraction. The border between perception and cognition is poorly defined, and the term *social cognition* is at any rate much more common in the literature. I acknowledge that I may be making too much of the distinction. But to me, perception and cognition have different shades of meaning and I find them useful in different situations.

One way to get at the distinction between perception and cognition is through illusions. Figure 7.1 shows an example of the well-known Muller-Lyer illusion. Here the two horizontal lines are actually the same length—measure them and see for yourself—but the upper one looks much longer. Cognitively, you know that Line A is the same length as Line B. Perceptually, you cannot help seeing unequal lengths. In this illusion, perception and cognition are rather starkly dissociable.

Can the same dissociation be demonstrated in the social realm? Is it possible to perceive awareness to be present in a source that, cognitively, you know is incapable of it?

Ventriloquism is a good example of this distinction between social perception and social cognition. The most obvious component of ventriloquism is a simple auditory–visual illusion in which the sound of the voice seems to come from the puppet's moving lips. But this so-called visual-capture illusion is mere surface and distracts from the deeper illusion of ventriloquism. When you see a good ventriloquist pick up a puppet and the puppet looks around, reacts, and talks, you experience an illusion of an intelligent mind that is directing its awareness here and there. Ventriloquism is a social illusion.

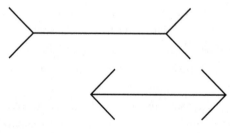

FIGURE 7.1

Which horizontal line is longer? They are the same length in the well-known Muller-Lyer illusion.

As a member of the audience you know cognitively, intellectually, that the puppet has no independent mind, but you fall for the illusion anyway. You have an impression of awareness emanating from the puppet. This phenomenon suggests that your brain constructs a perception-like model of the puppet's attentional state. The model provides you with the information that awareness is present and has a source inside the puppet. The model is automatic, meaning that you cannot choose to block it from occurring. If you watch the puppet show, you will get the impression. With a good ventriloquist who knows how to move the puppet in realistic ways, to direct its gaze with good timing, to make it react to its environment in a plausible way—with the right cues that tickle your system in the right way—the effect pops out. The puppet seems to come alive and seems to be aware of its world.

Puppetry therefore nicely illustrates three points. First, we construct models of other minds. Second, along with many other aspects of mind, we attribute the property of awareness to other people. Third, that model of awareness that we construct and attribute to somebody else is more perceptual in nature than cognitive. When interacting with another person, we have an impression of an awareness physically originating in that person.

Perceiving Awareness in Someone Else and in Oneself

Figure 7.2 illustrates the proposed relationship between awareness and attention. I'll explain the relationship first in the context of a person (Abel) perceiving somebody else's (Bill's) attention. Then I'll generalize the explanation to include the perception of one's own attention.

In this figure, Abel looks at Bill and Bill looks at a coffee cup. First consider Bill, whose visual attention is focused on the cup. Neuroscience is now able to provide a fairly detailed account of visual attention. One stimulus representation in the brain wins a

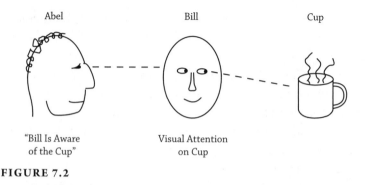

FIGURE 7.2

Awareness as a model of attention. Bill's visual attention is directed at the cup. Abel, observing Bill, constructs a model of Bill's mental state. Part of that model is the construct that Bill is aware of the cup. In this formulation, awareness is a construct that represents the attentional state of a brain.

neuronal competition among other representations. Bill's visual system builds a representation of the coffee cup, and that representation wins the attentional competition.

Now consider Abel, whose machinery for social perception constructs a model of Bill's mind. This type of model-building is called "theory of mind."[6] Able constructs a theory of Bill's mind. This model probably includes many attributes, such as Bill's possible thoughts, emotions, beliefs, and desires. Abel may have a rather rich model of Bill's mind. At least some part of that model concerns Bill's state of attention. Abel's model of Bill's attention includes the following three complex chunks of information. First, awareness is present. Second, the awareness originates from Bill. Third, the awareness is directed toward the cup. These properties—the property of awareness and its source and target—are bound together into a representation in Abel's brain.

In this formulation, Bill's visual attention is an event in the world to be perceived, and awareness is the perceptual counterpart to it constructed by Abel's social machinery. Note the distinction between the reality (Bill's attentional process) and the perceptual model of the reality (Abel's perception that Bill is aware). The reality includes the physics of light entering the eye, the body orientation and gaze direction of Bill, and a large set of hidden neuronal processes in Bill's brain. The perceptual model of that reality describes an amorphous, somewhat ethereal property of awareness that can be spatially localized at least vaguely to Bill and that, in violation of the physics of optics, emanates from Bill toward the object of his awareness and somehow takes possession of that object. The perceptual model is schematic, implausible from the point of view of physics, but useful for keeping track of Bill's state and therefore for helping to predict Bill's behavior. As in all perception, the perceptual model of awareness is useful rather than accurate.

Consider now the modified situation in which Abel and Bill are the same person. We are always in a social context because we always perceive and interact with ourselves. Abel/Bill focuses visual attention on the coffee cup. Abel/Bill also constructs a model of the attentional process. The model includes the following complex chunks of information: awareness is present, the awareness emanates from me, the awareness is directed at the cup.

If asked, "Are you aware of the cup?" Abel/Bill's brain can scan the contents of this model and answer, "Yes."

If asked, "What exactly do you mean by your awareness of the cup?" Abel/Bill's brain can again scan the informational model, abstract properties from it, and on the basis of that information report something like, "My awareness is a feeling, a vividness, an experience, a mental seizing of the stimulus such that I can now choose to react to it. My awareness is located inside me. In a sense it *is* me. It is my mind apprehending something. But the awareness is also linked to the cup. The color, the shape, all of these attributes of the cup have associated with them the property of my being aware of them." These summaries reflect the brain's quirky and complex model of the process of attending to something.

The example of Abel, Bill, and the coffee cup focuses on visual attention and visual awareness. The concept, however, is general.

Bill could just as well attend to a coffee cup, a sound, a smell, a feeling, a thought, a movement intention, a recalled memory, or many other cognitive, emotional, and sensory events. In the present theory, awareness is a reconstructed model of attention, and thus anything that can be the subject of attention can also be the subject of awareness.

Tracking Someone Else's Eyes

One of the primary ways we track someone's attention is by watching the eyes. And humans have unusual eyes. The contrast between the dark iris and white sclera is greater than for most other species. One possible explanation for the unusual contrast is that it is an evolutionary adaptation to allow humans to monitor each other's gaze.[7] When people scan a picture of a face, we tend to look disproportionately more at the eyes, as though seeking information from that facial feature.[8] People are excellent at detecting even tiny changes in someone's gaze direction.[9] We are experts at watching other people's eyes and extracting information from eyes.

A possible brain mechanism for social attention was discovered in the 1980s by Perrett and colleagues.[3] They were studying the monkey brain, monitoring the activity of neurons in a region of the cortex called the superior temporal sulcus (STS). The animal was shown pictures of eyes. Some neurons became active in response to pictures of eyes that looked to the left, others to pictures of eyes that looked to the right. A special machinery in the monkey brain seemed to be dedicated to the task of tracking someone else's gaze.

Further experiments using human volunteers in a brain scanner showed that the human brain also contained a specialized machinery for tracking someone else's gaze.[2,4,5,10]

The idea of social attention was elaborated by many scientists. One of the more interesting accounts was proposed in 1995 by Baron-Cohen.[1] In his account, the ability to reconstruct someone else's thoughts begins with the EDD as he called it, the eye direction detector. The EDD provides crucial information to other proposed modules in the brain, including the intentionality detector and the theory of mind mechanism. One of his more influential proposals was the shared attention mechanism. This proposed mechanism detects when you and someone else near you are paying attention to the same thing. It is radar for social alignment.

But do we really align our attention with other people's? Do we have a natural herd instinct when it comes to attention, pointing our eyes collectively at the same thing as a means of social cohesion or social communication?

Posner introduced a now famous task for studying human attention.[11] In that task, which is diagrammed in Figure 7.3A, you look at the center of a display screen. At an unpredictable time a small spot, the target, appears either to the left or the right. As soon as the target appears, you must press a button as quickly as possible. Sometimes the location of the target is precued. A square is briefly flashed on the screen, and then shortly thereafter the target appears at that same location. In these cases, your reaction time is significantly faster. Your spatial attention has been directed by the cue to the correct location, speeding up your processing of the target spot. In contrast, sometimes the cue is presented on one side and then, shortly thereafter, the target is presented on the opposite side. In those cases, your reaction time is slower. Your spatial attention has been diverted by the cue to the wrong side, thereby slowing your ability to detect the target. This elegant paradigm has become a staple method to study spatial attention.

Friesen and Kingstone[12] used a clever modification of the task, diagrammed in Figure 7.3B. In this task, you look at a drawing of a face in the center of a display screen. The eyes on the face may suddenly look to the left or to the right. A fraction of a second later a target spot appears either to the left or to the right. Your task is to press a button as quickly as possible to indicate the appearance of the target stimulus. In this paradigm, the direction of gaze of the

(A)   Posner Task with Standard Cue

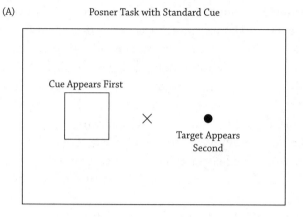

(B)   Posner Task with Gaze Cue

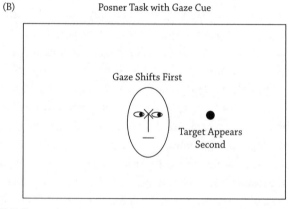

FIGURE 7.3

Testing visual attention with the Posner task. (A) In the standard version, a person looks at the central cross. Then a square cue flashes briefly, drawing attention to one location. Then a target dot flashes briefly. The person must press a button as soon as the target appears. When the cue draws attention away from the location of the target, the person responds slowly. When the cue draws attention toward the location of the target, the person responds quickly. In this way, visual attention can be demonstrated. (B) In the social attention version, the cue that draws attention is not a square around a location but a picture of a face that looks toward one side or the other.

central face acts as an attentional cue. When the face looks to the left and the target then appears on the left, your reaction time is shorter, indicating that your attention followed the face's gaze shift to the left. When the face looks to the right and then the target appears on the left, your reaction time is longer, indicating that your attention initially followed the face's gaze shift to the right and then had to shift back to the target on the left.

In this task, you are not told to follow the gaze of the face. You are given no instructions at all about the eyes on that face. But you evidently can't help shifting your attention in the direction that the face is looking. This finding was initially interpreted as evidence for a special mechanism in the human brain that monitors the gaze of others and aligns attention between people. Where you see someone else looking, your own attention automatically follows.

It is only fair to report a body of work that, on the whole, has ambiguous findings. Other scientists tried to replicate this effect of gaze in the Posner task.[13-15] The results were mixed. Gaze direction was not unique. A simple arrow at the center of the screen pointing to the right or left, or a dot stepping to the right or left, had a similar ability to direct people's attention. Eyes looking to the right or left were not special. Some have argued that a gaze cue may be more potent in drawing attention than a nongaze cue,[16] but by and large the evidence suggests that any cue will draw attention.

These results represent a failure to find any special effect of gaze monitoring. A person's attention does, indeed, tend to automatically follow the direction of someone else's gaze. But it also automatically follows any number of other cues and pointers. The results using the Posner task have tended to put a damper on the hypothesis of a special mechanism for social attention.

I believe that the pessimism is unwarranted. The limit of the Posner task, and also its strength, is that it can generalize across different kinds of cues. If a red square suddenly turns green, it will draw attention to its region of space. If a stationary square suddenly jiggles, that jiggle will also draw attention to its region of space.

Clearly, color and motion are not the same thing. They are processed by different circuitry in the visual system. Nobody would argue on the basis of the Posner task that the brain utterly lacks separate, specialized mechanisms for color and motion. Yet in the Posner task, color and motion function in a similar way. They cannot easily be disentangled. The task is therefore not the right tool to distinguish one perceptual mechanism from another. The fact that a pair of eyes moving to the left or right draws attention but that an arrow pointing to the left or right also draws attention just as well says little or nothing about the brain's specialized mechanism for processing eyes. These particular studies neither refute nor support the hypothesis of social attention.

I've described these complexities and mixed results for the sake of accuracy and completeness. The literature does contain some controversy. I do not wish to simplify or ignore the inconvenient details. However, taken together, the evidence on gaze and the brain point toward a particular conclusion. The human brain (and the monkey brain) seems to be equipped with specialized machinery that monitors the gaze of others.

Does the Attention Schema Theory Equate Awareness with an Eye Tracker?

In talking about the attention schema theory with colleagues and friends, I encounter scientific interest, enthusiasm, and inevitably some disagreement. The counterarguments tend to cluster into a few common forms. Throughout this book I address these common counterarguments. Here I would like to address what is probably the most common criticism of the attention schema theory.

According to the theory, awareness is a reconstructed model of attention. We often know where someone is attending by observing where someone's eyes are pointing. Therefore the theory (according to this criticism) equates awareness with eye tracking. But how can awareness be explained as an eye tracker? A simple machine, available on the market for the past few decades, uses infrared light bounced off of the cornea to track eye position. Point the device at a person and it can determine where the person is looking. The device is far more accurate, actually, than a human observer. Does the eye tracker perceive consciousness in the person whose eyes it is tracking? Of course it doesn't. If you put fake eyeballs on a machine and attach an eye tracker to that same machine such that it can track its own eye position, does that mean the machine has become a conscious being? No. Therefore, the theory must be wrong.

I find this criticism to be superficial because it so obviously misunderstands the theory. I believe the origin of the criticism lies in the social-attention literature, in which essentially all work is devoted to the issue of the eyes. How does one person know where another person is looking? The experiments described in the previous section focus entirely on how person A monitors the gaze of person B. The idea has gotten into the scientific culture that social attention is a matter of computing a gaze vector. Baron-Cohen's proposed mechanism is after all the eye direction detector (EDD). The concept has fossilized into an acronym.

Given this prevailing bias, perhaps it is easy for scientists to misunderstand the attention schema theory. It may be easy to mistake the attention schema itself for a mere eye tracker. How can an eye tracker, an eye direction detector, be responsible for awareness?

It isn't. Eye tracking is too narrow an understanding of the attention schema.

Eye position is certainly a useful cue for reconstructing someone's attentional state. Consider, however, two blind people talking to each other. By voice, by emotional nuance, by the implicit and explicit message of the words, each one is able to reconstruct something about the other person's attention. What thought is the other attending to? What idea? What sound? What emotion lies at the current center of attention? What does it mean to pay attention, in terms of deeper processing and impact on behavior? No eye tracking is occurring.

In the present theory, eye tracking is not necessary. It is merely a useful peripheral cue. It may be a dominant cue, but without it other sensory cues can stand in. The sensory cues themselves are not at the center of the theory. What is important is the rich informational representation of attentional state that is constructed on the basis of the cues.

In the attention schema theory, the human brain constructs a model of what it *means* to pay attention to something. An eye tracker, alas, does no such thing. It merely registers that a person's eyes are pointed in a particular direction.

In Chapter 5, I compared the attention schema to the body schema. Students who are new to thinking about the body schema sometimes make a similar mistake: they confuse the body schema for a registry of joint angles. Sensors in the joints can detect joint angle. By pooling information from many joints, you could track the body's configuration and movement. But this simple sensory tracking is not the same as a body schema. The body schema pulls together information from many sources—sensors in the joints, vision of the arm, expectation, prior knowledge about the structure of the body, and so on. On the basis of that converging information, a simulation of the body is constructed. The simulation can be used to understand and predict the physical consequences of movement.

Similarly, we do indeed track eye position in other people and also in ourselves. Eye position is one clue to one aspect of attention. It can help inform the attention schema. But the attention schema should not be confused with an eye tracker.

Probing the Attention Schema with a Picture

In psychology, when a mental trait is proposed, one way to define it more precisely is to find a test that probes for it. Can we find a test

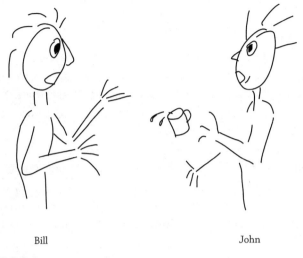

Bill   John

FIGURE 7.4

A cartoon to help demonstrate the attention schema. Given a story to explain the situation in the cartoon, you are able to intuitively understand the attentional states of the characters.

such that, if you have an attention schema, you can answer the questions correctly, and if you don't you can't?

In the cartoon in Figure 7.4, Bill and John are looking at each other in apparent shock while John drops a cup of coffee. Consider some questions about the picture.

Question 1

Is Bill's gaze directed toward John's face or toward John's hand?

This question asks explicitly about the direction of gaze. If you answer a question of this nature, you might activate your attention schema, but the answer does not strictly *require* any sophisticated understanding of attention. It requires only a geometric computation. Much of the research on social attention focuses on the low-level task of computing the direction of gaze and therefore misses the more interesting substance of the attention schema.

Question 2

Is Bill angry?

This question requires you to reconstruct someone else's mental state. In answering the question you might use facial cues to guess at Bill's emotions. But you are not specifically asked about Bill's attentional state. You are not required to use an attention schema to answer the question.

It would be wrong, however, to assume that an attention schema is definitely not recruited. Depending on the strategy you use, you might very well rely on an attention schema. One way to answer the question is to figure out which object is in Bill's attention and then to determine whether that object might make somebody angry. In that approach to answering the question, you are indeed using at least some inner knowledge of attention.

This example demonstrates how difficult it is to cleanly separate mental processes. A question, even one that seems simple, might tap into a variety of complex processes.

Question 3

Imagine a back-story. Bill and John are in the park talking about a news item that they both heard on the radio that morning. Apparently, a Siberian tiger escaped from the local zoo and is roving the neighborhood. Suddenly they hear a tiger roaring loudly from the bushes directly behind Bill. The picture shows their immediate reactions.

At the particular moment captured in the picture, is Bill more aware of the tiger behind him or of the coffee spill in front of him?

In this case, where Bill is looking has nothing to do with the object of his attention. He is looking at John, but he is probably attending to the noisy tiger behind him. A basic knowledge of the dynamics of attention is required to answer the question. Signals in the brain compete with each other, and the signal with the biggest boost will tend to outcompete and suppress other signals. People attend to salient sensory stimuli, especially dangerous stimuli, and the most salient stimulus present, the tiger roar, will probably outcompete other stimuli. Even a coffee spill, normally an attention-grabbing event, will probably be outcompeted by the tiger roar. In the heat of the moment, Bill may be entirely unaware of the coffee spill. To answer the question, you do not need to plod through these reasons explicitly. You certainly don't need to know anything about how signals compete in the brain. Your knowledge about attention is implicit. You understand the dynamics of attention intuitively. You can even guess Bill's likely reactions. Whatever his actions will be, they will be driven by the tiger, not the spilled coffee. He is unlikely to kneel down and help John mop up the spill. He is more likely to run. Your implicit understanding of attention includes a rather sophisticated grasp of its competitive dynamics and an understanding of how attention affects behavior. Here we have tapped into the attention schema and clearly separated it from the low-level task of eye tracking.

The many examples in this chapter and the previous chapters—not just those involving Bill and John and the spilled coffee but also illusions of other people's gaze fixed on us from behind, the fad of mesmerism, the strange persistence of the extromission account of vision, the potent sense of awareness that emanates from a ventriloquist's puppet, and so on—indicate that when we observe others, when we think about other people, among the many aspects of mind and emotion that we reconstruct is attentional state. We intuitively understand the dynamics and behavioral consequences of attention, and we perceive it as awareness originating in other agents.

8

How Do I Distinguish My Awareness from Yours?

In the previous chapters I suggested that your own private awareness and your ability to attribute awareness to someone else are products of the same machinery in your brain, the machinery for social perception. That machinery computes the property of awareness and can attribute it to you or to others.

Yet why does your own awareness come with such internal vividness, whereas the awareness you attribute to someone else is so much dimmer? Clearly the process of constructing your own awareness cannot be precisely the same as constructing someone else's awareness. When you look at a green apple you experience a vivid consciousness of green. When John looks at a green apple and you are observing him, you may note that he is aware of the apple, you may even get the impression of an awareness emanating from him, but you do not reconstruct his vivid consciousness of green in the same way that you construct your own. You do not feel privy to John's experience.

Here I offer five speculations to explain the difference in constructing your own awareness and attributing awareness to someone else. All five of these speculations are extrapolations from, applications of, or interpretations of, the attention schema theory. They are not rival explanations. All five might contribute. They are, however, speculations and should be taken with some reasonable skepticism.

Richer and More Continuous Information about Yourself

In the present theory, you construct a model of your own awareness and a model of John's awareness. Your model of your own awareness, let us call it *A1*, is based on a rich set of internally accessible information that is continuously present. Your model of John's awareness, let us call it *A2*, is based on limited observation and relies on imperfect cues such as gaze direction, facial expression, and body posture. It may be, therefore, that *A1* is simply a more robust, more detailed, or more strongly activated representation than *A2*, much as, for example, the sound of your own voice is inevitably more resonant and richer than the sound of someone else's voice.

Interaction with Somatosensory Processing

In Chapter 6 I discussed the possible link between awareness and somatosensory processing. Mentally focusing on a part of the body can prime the sense of touch, in effect making you more sensitive in that body part.[1] The assignment of *A1*, your model of your own awareness, to a location inside your own body could cause this type of priming. It could subtly activate the processing of body-related sensory signals. That added component may contribute to making *A1* more "vivid" or "present" than *A2*. *A1* might come with a subtle enhancement of touch or pressure, whereas *A2*, assigned to a distant location, does not.

Awareness of Someone Else's Awareness

In the present theory, you can construct a model of someone else's attentional state (assigning awareness to someone else), and you can also construct a model of your own attentional state (assigning awareness to yourself). The two models may depend on similar neuronal machinery, but they are two different chunks of information. If you construct a model of someone else's attentional state, then in no sense are you yourself aware of it. You have assigned the property of awareness to the other person, not to yourself. In the present hypothesis, to process someone else's attentional state, thus to assign awareness to someone else, and at the same time to be aware that you are doing it requires an extra layer. It requires a model of how your own attentional state is focused on someone else's attentional state. It requires the compound, bound set of information:

[I] [am aware] [John is aware].

By the logic of the attention schema theory, much of the attribution of awareness to other people may well occur outside of one's own consciousness. The attention schema theory makes a distinction between constructing your own awareness, constructing a model of someone else's awareness, and constructing your own awareness that someone else is aware.

The Importance of Personal Perspective

You and John are both looking at an apple. Your brain contains three relevant chunks of information. The first is information that represents your own awareness, $A1$. The second is your reconstruction of John's awareness, $A2$. The third is visual information, V, that represents the apple. Which of these chunks of information will be bound together into a single, larger representation? Will you construct $A1 + V$, or $A2 + V$?

The difficulty with $A2 + V$ is that it contains incompatible spatial information. $A2$, your model of John's awareness, contains a spatial structure in which awareness has a source inside John. The visual information, V, however, is perspective specific. It is information about the apple as seen from your spatial perspective. The two chunks of information, $A2$ and V, are not compatible with each other.

You would not normally perceive a red house to be yellow just because a yellow car is nearby. Your visual system would not normally bind together features that mismatch in location. In the same manner, in the present speculation, you would not bind together $A2$ and V because of the mismatch in spatial structure. In contrast, the two chunks of information $A1$ and V are mutually compatible. $A1$ is a model of awareness attributed to your own location, and V is visual information about an apple as seen from your own spatial location. The natural conjunction to construct would be $A1 + V$.

As a result, in this speculation, your brain constructs two representations. One is a larger, bound representation, $A1 + V$, the representation that defines your conscious experience of the green apple. When you introspect, that is, make decisions about the properties of that data set, you are able to report that you are looking at an apple and that it has a set of properties attached to it including color, shape, location in space, and your awareness of it. The awareness, the experienceness, is bound to the visual information. It acts like color. It acts like a perceptual feature bound to the other features that define the apple.

The second representation is $A2$, a representation that is not bound to specific visual properties. This second representation describes a somewhat ethereal, invisible stuff of intelligence or of mental energy or of experience that is inside John and that is emanating out of him toward the apple.

In this speculation, your brain constructs your own awareness (a model of your own attentional state) just as it constructs an awareness for John (a model of John's attentional state). The two models are similar in nature. They are both models of intelligent, attentive processing. They both depend on the same underlying neuronal machinery. The difference between them is that the awareness that you construct for yourself is tightly bound to the sensory information about the apple, whereas the awareness that you construct for John is not.

Resonance

If the present theory is correct, then awareness is the brain's way to represent attention. But attention is the process of enhancing a representation. The consequence is a resonance loop. Your own awareness, in this theory, is locked in a positive feedback loop with your own attention. The two boost each other. One affects the other; the other affects the one. The brain's representation of something and the something that is being represented blend together.

In contrast, in constructing a model of someone else's attentional state, no such resonance exists. The loop is open rather than closed. You may construct a model of John's attention, but that model in your brain will have no direct effect on his attention, and his attention will not directly operate on your brain's models.

In the attention schema theory, this property of resonance may be the most profound difference between constructing your own awareness and constructing an awareness that you attribute to someone else. The two processes may be similar and may rely on similar mechanisms in the brain, but they should not be equated with each other. In this theory, constructing your own awareness necessarily has a different dynamic.

Failures of the System: Group Consciousness

If the speculations above are correct, if distinguishing your awareness from John's awareness is a matter of the subtleties of computation, then errors in those computations should occur at least some of the time. Earlier in this chapter, I gave the example of a yellow car next to a red house. You would not normally perceive the house to be yellow. But the fact is that, occasionally, the visual system makes mistakes of exactly this sort—false conjunctions. If you glance at the scene and pay it little attention, you are prone to make that type of error. Similarly, in the social domain, in the process of constructing models of minds, a brain might make false conjunctions. For example, it should be possible on occasion to construct the false conjunction of $A1 + A2$, joining your model of your own awareness with your model of John's awareness. In that case, you are constructing a false informational model in which a single awareness is shared by you and someone else. This false conjunction is tantamount to a consciousness illusion.

Consider again the case of you and John looking at an apple. The visual information about the apple is perspective specific. It is consistent with your own perspective and inconsistent with John's perspective. You see the apple from the perspective of your own gaze and your own location in the world and so bind it to a model of your own mind, not to a model of John's mind. But now consider a different item: an emotion (E) such as embarrassment or joy. An emotion does not have a specific visual perspective. It does not have the same spatial or directional clues that clearly associate it with your particular location in the world. If the present speculations are correct, then you should tend more often to confuse who exactly is experiencing the emotion. When feeling joyful, you might tend incorrectly to attribute joyfulness to others nearby. When watching someone make an embarrassing gaff, you might not know precisely who is more embarrassed, you or the other person. If you incorrectly bind $A1 + E$ and, at the same time, $A2 + E$, attributing the same emotional feature to two models of awareness, then you have in effect constructed the compound and nonsensical representation of $A1 + A2 + E$. You have bound $A1$ and $A2$ into the same larger representation.

That false conjunction is tantamount to group consciousness—the illusion that you are joined to other people's awareness, that you share a single awareness with the company around you, with a mob like the famous shared-consciousness party crowd at Woodstock, with a spouse you've come to know so well that you feel as though you are sharing his or her thoughts, or with a good friend, a comrade who has passed through intense emotional experiences with you. This sort of nonstandard consciousness, the joining of awareness, comes straight from the world of alternative spirituality and pseudoscience and makes no sense in traditional views of consciousness. If consciousness is an emergent state of the brain, if it is a feeling generated by the information in your brain, then how can two people share it? How can the consciousness from your brain merge with the consciousness from John's brain? The claim must be myth or silliness. People must be making it up. There is no mechanism for people to experience consciousness in that way.

Yet, in the attention schema theory, although you cannot literally share someone else's awareness, you can have the illusion. Because awareness is *described* by the brain rather than produced, because it is a chunk of information constructed by the brain, it is always possible for the brain to construct a nonstandard or dysfunctional model. Experiences that may seem scientifically anathema, such as the experience of a shared consciousness, or an out-of-body experience in which one's consciousness seems to float free of the body, or multiple personality disorder in which many conscious agents seem to exist in the same head—all of these experiences are extremely hard to explain if consciousness is truly an ethereal feeling that emerges from the brain in the traditional view. But they are easy to explain if consciousness is computed information—if it is a rich, complex description constructed by the brain. Altered states of consciousness are simply altered versions of the descriptive model.

Failures of the System: Multiple Personalities

The multiple personality disorder, or the dissociative identity disorder as it is officially called, is characterized by a set of different conscious minds, each with its own personality, present in the same brain.[2] Some patients have only two identities and others have many. There is considerable disagreement about whether it is a real disorder that arises naturally or whether it is the result of therapists inadvertently conveying expectations and convincing their patients to act in that manner.

To have different personalities in the same brain is normal. We all have that condition. At home, in one context, with my five-year-old son, I act one way. At work, in another context, I behave in a different way. A forty-year-old man visits his high school buddies and slips into an adolescent personality. A woman switches from a motherly personality to a tough business personality.

The dissociative identity disorder is different from normal social behavior in two key ways. One is that the different personalities have separate memories. When Fred is expressed, he can't remember events or has a hazy memory of events that took place when George was in control.

A second characteristic is that the personalities switch in sudden phase transitions. The transition is rapid; two personalities do not generally overlap in their control. These switches are not always under the voluntary will of the patient. Somehow one personality wins out and pops to the top, and then, after a while, another personality wins.

The symptomology is so sensational that it has rather strained the credulity of many scientists, clinicians, and trial juries. Patients are often simply not believed. The condition probably occurs at a higher rate than is reported, given how stigmatized it is and how often it is disregarded as made-up nonsense or as a convenient excuse for bad behavior.

One probable reason for the skepticism is that, although our culture has a mix of many different views on consciousness, most of these views are incompatible with having more than one consciousness in the same head. In religious views of consciousness, a spirit occupies the space inside us; in which case suddenly developing more than one spirit is nonsensical or perhaps even heretical. For people who have naturalistic views of consciousness, the typical view is that consciousness arises from the functioning of the brain; in which case, again, it is difficult to understand how two inner feelings can arise from the functioning of the same brain, or why the two experiences would take turns controlling the body. Multiple personality disorder is simply inconsistent with most commonly held theories of consciousness.

But what about the attention schema theory? Does it at least allow for the theoretical possibility of multiple personalities? If awareness itself is a model constructed by the brain, then the possibility of several models competing with each other, alternating in phase transitions, is not only theoretically possible but also predicted. That condition should occur at least sometimes in some people.

The notion that two perceptual models might compete and alternate with each other is well accepted. Examples abound. In the famous Necker cube, for example, as you look at a wire frame cube, sometimes one surface seems to be in front and sometimes the other seems to be. The image itself is consistent with both perceptions, thus the two perceptions switch in what is called a bistable manner. The brain can construct two different models to account for the visual data, the two models are incompatible with each other, and therefore the two compete. In that competition, sometimes one model wins and suppresses its rival, sometimes the other pops to the top. You can partly influence the phase transitions by staring at one part of the image or another, but the transitions occur somewhat randomly.

The phase transitions in the dissociative personality disorder are so suspiciously like the phase transitions of bistable perception that they provide rather suggestive evidence that awareness is a constructed, perception-like model.

I am not certain that I want to go on record as championing the dissociative identity disorder. Perhaps many cases are faked, or mistaken, or misdiagnosed. But I do suggest that the disorder is not nonsensical. It *ought* to happen, at least sometimes, at least to some people. If the present theory of consciousness is correct, then a brain should be able to construct two competing awarenesses, two models, each with its own associations, memories, and emotional traits that are linked to it, and the models should compete with each other, resulting in phase transitions in which one or the other pops to the top and takes over.

9

Some Useful Complexities

When a person says, "I am aware of X," that statement is of course a verbal summary. It is an abstraction. It is shorthand for a much richer set of information that lies deeper in the brain. Each word has so much meaning behind it that it is like a flag that stands for an entire country. In this final chapter of Part 1, I explore some of the detail and complexity. Just how many separable components make up the construct, "I am aware of X," and which components are essential for awareness itself?

The information "I am aware of X" could be labeled as C, the information set that encompasses my conscious mind at the moment. Moment by moment, C changes as new items enter or fade from my consciousness.

C can be broken into three large, complicated chunks of information.

One chunk is information on the nature of "I." Many theories of consciousness have focused on this understanding of oneself as an entity, proposing essentially that self-knowledge is the same thing as consciousness. Let us term this chunk of information S, for self.

Another chunk of information describes the properties of X, the thing about which I am aware. Many theories of consciousness have focused on the brain's processing of X. Theories of visual consciousness, for example, almost all focus on the visual processing of visual information in the visual system.

A third chunk of information depicts the meaning of "am aware of." In the present theory the brain constructs an attention schema, a rich informational model that depicts the dynamics of a brain attending to something. Let us label this chunk of information A.

The information "I am aware of X" is an integration of all three components: $S + A + X$.

The formula can be broken down into finer chunks. The depiction of me as an entity, S, contains subcomponents. For example, some of the information that defines me is about me as a physical being with a specific location, body structure, movement capability, and ownership of my limbs. This part of S is my body schema. Let us call it PS, for physical self.

Another set of information that defines me is more psychological in nature. It is the vast collection of information that I have about myself as a mental being with certain feelings, thoughts, and personality patterns. Let us call this information set MS, for mental self.

Yet another source of information that my brain has on myself as a person is autobiographical memory. At any moment, I may have specific memories active in my brain, supplying me with a sense of my own history and my own trajectory through life. Let us call this information set RS, for the recalled memories related to the self.

The information set A also contains subcomponents. As I discussed in Chapter 6, the human brain tends to construct a spatial embodiment for awareness. My awareness is assigned a location, a perspective, and can even seem to flow fluid-like through space and time. Let us term this part of the information set PA, for the physical properties attributed to awareness.

The information set A also contains a description of mental attributes. We report awareness as an intelligence, a private experience, a knowing, a mental seizing of something. Let us term this part of the information set MA, for the more mental or experiential properties of awareness.

The final part of the formula, X, the depiction of the object of awareness, can also contain subcomponents. The representation of an apple, for example, is a collection of information about shape, color, location, motion, texture, and so on. Other objects of awareness, whether external objects or internal events, may break down along other lines.

We now have a much more complex, subdivided formula, from

$$C$$

to

$$S + A + X$$

to

$$PS + MS + RS + PA + MA + X.$$

This neat division is, of course, solely for intellectual convenience. The reality must be messier, a juggling of many more components and subcomponents that change over time, that in some cases are distinct from each other and in other cases grade into each other. But the formal diagramming of components provides at least a handle on the information that, in the attention schema theory, can be bound together to form consciousness. This massive set of information sprawls over much of the brain, interconnected by some mechanism of informational binding that is not yet fully understood (though I will talk more about it in Chapter 11). Collectively it is a single, coherent description. It is a representation of a state. Because it is a representation, because it is information, cognitive machinery can access it, summarize its properties, and on that basis decide and report, "X is so; it has this and that property; moreover, the property of awareness is attached to X; in particular, I experience X; I have an inner feeling of X; I, the aware being, have thoughts and feelings and personhood; I exist here, in this physical instantiation and mental condition; it is this physical and mental being that has an awareness of X."

In short form: "I am aware of X."

Where in these many components is awareness? A holistic answer might reasonably be that all of this information put together—

information that depicts me as a physical being, information that depicts me as a mental being, information that depicts the act of awareness, information that depicts X itself—composes consciousness.

A more dissected answer might be that awareness, awareness itself, the pure essence of it, is specifically the component MA. It is the representation of experienceness. It is the brain's depiction of the relationship between the knower and the known.

Either approach might do—the more holistic or the more dissected—but I find the more precise, dissected definition to be particularly useful. It refers to the essential part of the larger phenomenon.

Consider a thought experiment. Imagine removing chunks of information from consciousness one by one. Of the long string of proposed components, $PS + MS + RS + PA + MA + X$, what would happen as each component is erased? At what point would awareness itself disappear?

Is X necessary? Is it necessary to be aware of any specific information in order to be aware? Can you be aware, simply aware, without any target of the awareness? I have had conversations with colleagues, especially those who study visual consciousness, who scratch their heads and say, "What does that state even mean? I am aware of a color. I am aware of a shape. I am aware of a movement. But without any target of the awareness, how can I have any awareness? It's nonsensical." Speaking entirely subjectively, however, I think it is a common occurrence for me. I reach a state in which I seem to be aware, my brain must have constructed that particular feature, but I do not seem to have any specific item about which I am aware. I am simply an aware being. Maybe this state corresponds to my brain constructing $S + A$. I have constructed a model of myself as a being with an awareness, but the model is temporarily incomplete because it is not linked to any specific object of the awareness. It may seem nonsensical to be aware without being aware of something, but the brain can certainly construct an informational description that is nonsensical or incomplete.

What about MS, information about my mental self? When I am aware of something, does that awareness necessarily always imply an understanding that there is a mental "I" that is aware, complete with its own emotions, ideas, and beliefs? Undoubtedly, we humans fall into lapses when the brain simply does not compute much about the inner life. I would guess that yes, even failing for a moment to process that I am a mental or psychological agent, that I am *me*, I can still be aware of the world around me. Indeed, I would say much of my waking experience falls into this category: a simple, immediate, "animal" awareness of things and events around me. In that case, perhaps my system has constructed mainly $A + X$, without much of the S component represented.

It has been suggested that people have two modes of thinking, one in which awareness is inwardly focused and the other in which awareness is outwardly focused. Introspective awareness tends to activate its own distinct network of brain areas, the "default-mode network" as it is called.[1,2] Outwardly focused awareness tends to activate a greater range of brain regions. In the present theory, both modes of thinking involve an attention schema. Both involve awareness. But the two modes differ in the extent to which the attention schema, A, is linked to information about the self or information about external events. Inwardly focused awareness may be mostly a construction of $S + A$, and outwardly focused awareness may be mostly a construction of $A + X$.

What about RS, the recalled memories about myself? Suppose I suffer a Hollywood-style amnesia and have no memory of who I am or where I came from. Some essential part of my personhood, my consciousness, is gone. I am wiped clean. Many of my colleagues equate memory with consciousness. I don't deny the importance of auto-biographical memories. They help define the sense of self. They help make me *me*. But I would argue that they are not strictly necessary for awareness. Even if my memories were wiped, if I lost RS, I would still be *aware*. I would still be a conscious being, even if I no longer knew precisely who I was or how I came to be where I was.

What about PS, the representation of my physical self? Can I be conscious if, due to some processing lapse or brain trauma, I am unable to compute a body schema? Suppose I no longer understand that my limbs and torso are here, hinged and shaped this way and that way, or that these limbs belong to me personally. What does it mean to be aware of something, such as a thought, a sound, or a nearby object, and not know about myself as a physical thing to which the awareness can be anchored? I do not believe I have ever had that type of experience. I suspect the body schema is fairly robust and is more or less continuously computed. But I can imagine brain damage that might severely disrupt the body schema. In that case I would guess that, even in the absence of a sense of physical self, awareness is still possible, although it would be an unusual, altered type of awareness.

What about *PA*, the physical embodiment that is computed specifically for awareness, the information that awareness is located in my body, that it emanates from me? We already know that *PA* can be dysfunctional. In the out-of-body experience, awareness is assigned an incorrect point of origin and spatial perspective.[3,4] What would happen if I had no *PA*, if my model of awareness had no physical anchor? Suppose that, due to damage, my brain is no longer able to compute *PA*. My awareness is constructed as pure experienceness, timeless and spaceless, with no particular source or anchor in my body or anywhere else. I would guess that such a state is possible and qualifies as another unusual, altered type of awareness.

The only component left that seems, in this thought experiment, to be absolutely necessary for awareness is *MA*, the model of the mental attributes of awareness. In the attention schema theory, *MA* is information. It is a nuanced, rich description, the brain's way of describing to itself the essence of signal enhancement. Without *MA*, a brain has no basis to detect, conclude, report, process, assign a high degree of certainty to, or have anything else to do with awareness. *MA* defines experienceness. It defines awareness.

These thought experiments of separating one component from another are philosophically intriguing. But are any such manipulations possible in actuality? Can a brain compute the components separately? Certainly brain damage might take out one function or another, but can the normal healthy brain compute the components separately?

The theory makes a clear though subtle prediction: yes, the components can come apart. They can be computed in isolation, without binding one component to another. But they can come apart only in the absence of attention.

Attention does more than enhance one set of signals and suppress other, outcompeted signals. Attention has the effect of binding together the signals that have won the competition. Attention builds a single, unified representation. For example, when you pay attention to an apple, then the greenness, the roundness, and the motion of the apple are fused together into a single informational unit. Accessing one chunk of information necessarily also accesses the other chunks. When your attention is not focused on the apple, the features are not bound in that manner. The system can even become confused, and you may accidentally attribute the wrong color to an object. One of the properties of attention, therefore, is that it glues together disparate computed features. In the present theory, awareness is a computed feature. To bind it to another chunk of information requires attention.

It may be possible outside of attention, at the fringes of attention, or close to sleep to be aware, simply aware, without being aware of something, and without processing that you are the being who is aware. (One is reminded of some of the goal states of Buddhist meditation. Clear your mind of all thought. Achieve a pure awareness.)

Note that for such a state to occur, in the present theory, your brain must construct an attention schema, a model of attention, even though no focused attention is actually present. The model is incorrect. Certainly the brain can produce incorrect perceptual models. Such things happen. For example, in the absence of light entering the eye, the visual system computes representations that can be seen as dim floating colors and shapes. Likewise, in the absence of actual focused attention occurring in your brain, in theory the relevant circuitry should be able to construct a model of you directing a focused attention, and in theory that model is awareness, just awareness, unbound, unattached to a subject or an object, without a spatial or a temporal structure, without a location. Pure essence. Pure experienceness. But if you focus your attention on the question, or on anything else, on a nearby object, on your inner state, on a thought, on an emotion, then the binding should fall into place. At that moment, it is no longer possible to have awareness free floating, unattached to its subject or its object. The associations form and you become a specific agent aware of a specific set of objects or thoughts or emotions. In the attention schema theory, when you introspect to examine your own consciousness in an attentive, focused manner, you should get one type of picture. But if you let consciousness gather by itself, outside of attentive focus, you should obtain a different picture of it. Consciousness is something murky, complicated, contradictory, always changing. It may be that the attention schema theory has enough subtlety to account for so amorphous and mysterious a phenomenon.

The first half of this book explained the basic concepts of the attention schema theory. The theory is easily summarized. The brain uses a data-handling method, a common way in which signals interact, a process that neuroscientists call attention. The brain also constructs a constantly updated sketch, a schema, a rough model to describe that process of attention. That model is awareness. Because it is information, it is reportable. We can say that we have it. We can introspect and decide that we have it. The theory is rational, mechanistic, straightforward. Yet it also has emergent complexities. I've briefly outlined some of these complexities, including strange loops, resonance, and a great variety of altered states of consciousness. The underlying concepts may be simple, but the theory is not simplistic. The consciousness described by the theory sounds a great deal like the real thing.

So far I've said very little about how the attention schema theory might be implemented in specific regions of the brain. I've also said little about how the theory might mesh or conflict with previous theories of consciousness. The second half of the book addresses these topics.

PART TWO

COMPARISON TO PREVIOUS THEORIES AND RESULTS

10

Social Theories of Consciousness

The number and range of theories of consciousness that have been proposed—religious, philosophical, quantum mechanical, mystical, cellular, electrical, magnetic, computer-programmable, neuronal, psychological, social, cosmic, and metacosmic—is dizzying and inspires some degree of awe for human ingenuity. These theories tend to fall into categories, so that reviewing and discussing them is not an entirely hopeless task. However, I will leave that type of broad overview to other texts. For example, for an excellent summary of the consciousness literature, see Blackmore's account.[1]

In this second part of the book I take a selective look at the literature. I discuss previous theories and results that have a clear conceptual relevance to the attention schema theory. My interest lies in integrating the previous work with the present theory. I am not so much motivated to knock down previous views as to understand how they relate to each other and to the attention schema theory.

Despite this narrow filter on the literature, a very large range of perspectives and results are still covered here. These previous perspectives on consciousness include the relationship between consciousness and social intelligence, the relationship between consciousness and integrated information in the brain, the attempt to find neuronal circuits or responses in the brain that correlate with consciousness, the study of the partial loss of consciousness in severe brain damage, and the search for the neuronal machinery that allows humans to model and simulate other people's mind states. Within these broad categories, about twenty specific perspectives on consciousness are discussed and many more are mentioned.

I begin with two general approaches to consciousness. The attention schema theory shares strong similarities with both of these previous lines of thought. One approach is that consciousness is a product of our social capability. The second is that consciousness occurs when the information in the brain becomes highly interconnected.

These two approaches, the social approach and the integrated information approach, have little resemblance to each other. In some ways they are rivals. Each one has its advantages and its weaknesses. Yet in many ways they are both precursors to the present theory. The attention schema theory could be viewed as a way of drawing on the strengths of these two previous hypotheses while avoiding their weaknesses. In this chapter I discuss the social approach to consciousness, and in the next chapter I discuss the integrated information approach, in each case explaining how the attention schema theory builds on the previous work.

The Self-Narrative

We humans construct a narrative to explain other people's behavior. We constantly engage in social story-telling. So-and-so must be doing this or saying that because of a particular mood or agenda, a belief or reason. Do we use the same indirect process to construct a narrative of our own behavior? Perhaps we construct a self-narrative, a stream-of-consciousness account of ourselves, of our motives and reasons. Can a social narrative, turned inward, account for consciousness? This section describes some of the main social hypotheses about consciousness. Subsequent sections describe the most commonly noted difficulties with these theories.

In 1970, Gazzaniga[2] formulated one of the earliest examples of this approach to consciousness. He proposed that the human brain contains an "interpreter," a mechanism in the left hemisphere that constructs a verbal narrative to explain behavior.

Gazzaniga's proposal was based on experiments using split-brained patients. In order to control the spread of epilepsy, these patients underwent a surgical cut to the corpus callosum, the bundle of nerve fibers that connects one hemisphere to the other. After the surgery the two hemispheres were unable to communicate with each other directly. The left hemisphere was functionally isolated from the right. In these patients, therefore, it was possible to test the abilities of the two hemispheres separately. Since speech is generally controlled by the left hemisphere, anything the patient said was an indication of left-hemisphere thought. Yet the right hemisphere had enough linguistic skill to understand basic instructions and to act on them.

Gazzaniga's key experiment was to give instructions specifically to the right hemisphere of a patient, allow the subject to act out those instructions, and then ask the left hemisphere to explain why the patient had chosen to act in that way. For example, the right hemisphere might be instructed, "Point to your foot." The subject does so. How does the left hemisphere explain the behavior? The left, verbal hemisphere explains in words why that particular action was performed. But lacking any knowledge of the real reason, it makes up its own reason and seems confident in that confabulation. These split-brained subjects spun false, after-the-fact explanations of their own behavior with extraordinary confidence.

From this result Gazzaniga suggested that consciousness was essentially a tale that the brain tells itself to explain what it is doing and why it is doing it. He proposed that the left hemisphere contains something he called the interpreter, which spins explanatory stories about oneself as well as stories about other people.

This idea that consciousness is after-the-fact, that we make up a story to explain ourselves to ourselves, has cropped up many times in the literature in many variants. A similar proposal was made in 1977 by Nisbett and Wilson.[3] We tend to think of consciousness as a direct access to our own decisions, ideas, and thoughts. Yet Nisbett and Wilson suggested that, contrary to popular belief, the human brain has no privileged access to its own internal processes. We know about our mental states using the same tricks and inferences that we use to reconstruct the mental states of other people. We tell ourselves a story about ourselves. As a consequence, we routinely and confidently make up incorrect reasons for our own behavior.

Yet another variant of the same idea was proposed by Libet and colleagues.[4] These researchers focused on conscious choice—our sense of intentionality. We consciously choose to pick up a coffee cup, turn on a light, stand up, open a door, and so on. We all feel as though some inner consciousness first decided on how to act, and then having made the decision, directed our bodies to carry out the act. Conscious decision comes first, action comes second. Yet Libet and colleagues performed an experiment that suggested the order may be reversed. In that experiment, the action to be performed was simple. People were asked to press a button. They could press the button any time they wanted to. The choice was theirs. They watched the second hand on a clock and noted the precise time at which the thought, the intention to act, entered their minds. At the same time, the person had a set of electrodes placed on the scalp to monitor the electrical activity in the motor cortex, specifically in a region of the brain that plans movements of the finger.

The result of the experiment was counterintuitive. People confidently reported a particular time on the clock to be the instant, the key moment, when the conscious choice to act entered their heads. Yet the activity in the motor cortex consistently rose up a moment earlier. The order was backward. First motor cortex planned the action, then the conscious decision kicked in. By implication, the human brain chooses an action by means of unconscious processes. A different system in the brain then obtains information that the action is about to occur and constructs a story about how and why the act was intended. Consciousness, and in particular the conscious intention to act, is after-the-fact and indirect, as if we were observing ourselves and inferring our reasons.

This view of intentionality is controversial and may represent only a part of a more complex story.[5] In some instances the conscious intention comes first; in other instances it comes second. The story is not as simple as the original experiment suggested. Nonetheless, the experiment had an enormous impact on the way researchers thought about the problem. The experiment helped promote the view that consciousness is a narrative that the brain spins to make sense of what it is doing.

We certainly invent narratives to explain other people. But do we use the same brain machinery to explain ourselves? One way to get at this question is by a more direct measurement of brain activity, for example, by using a magnetic resonance imaging (MRI) scanner. Numerous studies, especially over the past ten years, have asked if the same brain areas are active when we think about other people and when we think about ourselves. When people are placed in an MRI scanner and asked to think about someone else's thoughts or emotions, a specific network of brain areas consistently lights up. Many of the same brain areas are also recruited when people are asked to monitor their own mental states.[6-10] These experiments lend support to the hypothesis of consciousness as a social construct, or at least to the hypothesis that some aspects of self-knowledge depend on the same machinery that is used to construct narratives about other people's minds.

The idea of the social construction of consciousness, that consciousness depends on high-level social cognition, or on people building up an understanding of how minds work, or on people thinking about thinking, has been elaborated and extended by many researchers. In some versions of the hypothesis, my consciousness is much larger than my understanding of myself. It is my understanding of the social context, the social universe in which I live and my own place in that larger context. In that way of thinking consciousness is a function of groups of people and is not really a private matter. It is not a function of a single brain but is an interactive medium, a kind of social web of information within which humans are embedded as we relate to each other.[11-13]

I have now described at least some of the main experiments and ideas about social theories of consciousness. They are quite diverse. They range from verbal stories of ourselves, such as Gazzaniga's interpreter, to conscious decisions that come after the fact, such as in the experiments of Libet and colleagues. They include experiments on networks of brain areas involved in social cognition, and they include some mind-bending speculations about consciousness as a group function instead of a property of individuals. Yet they all share certain characteristics. The social theories of consciousness share the following three properties.

First, the brain actively constructs an elaborate description or model or narrative about its own processing.

Second, that self-descriptive information is often wrong. The system that computes it has limited capacity and relies on limited cues.

Third, the machinery that computes the self-description is also used to compute explanations of other people. We understand ourselves and other people partly through the same means.

All three of these hypotheses are almost certainly correct. Given the range of experimental findings, it is hard to imagine how they could be wrong. However, the three properties by themselves do not necessarily explain the phenomenon of human consciousness. They may account for some of the contents of consciousness, especially some aspects of self-knowledge, but other aspects of consciousness are left unaddressed. The social theories of consciousness have notorious gaps.

The attention schema theory could be seen as a type of social theory of consciousness. The brain constructs a description or model of awareness and attributes it to other people. The same machinery also attributes awareness to oneself. The theory therefore borrows heavily from social approaches to consciousness. Yet because of the specifics of the theory, it avoids some of the standard pitfalls. In each of the following sections, I discuss a specific, common criticism of the social approach to consciousness. I also discuss how the attention schema theory might be able to add usefully to the approach, fill in some missing pieces, and avoid the same criticisms.

Self-Awareness versus Awareness in General

All of the social theories of consciousness described in the previous section focus on knowledge about mental events such as what emotions one is feeling, what thoughts one is having, and especially one's personal reasons for performing this or that action. Why did I choose to stand up and walk here? Why did I choose to say what I said? Why did I eat a cookie instead of a banana? The social theories of consciousness focus on the narrative that I use to explain my actions to myself. All of these mental processes—choices, thoughts, and emotions—are important, but they involve internal events only. The social theories of consciousness leave unaddressed the consciousness of external events. Of course, the brain constructs a narrative to explain its own behavior and its own thoughts. The hypothesis is sound. But how does that narrative relate to the raw sensory experience of, say, green, or pain, or the sound of G above middle C? Social theories tackle the question of self-awareness, not awareness in general.

The attention schema theory neatly solves this nagging problem of the social theories of consciousness.

Like other social approaches, the attention schema theory is about the brain reconstructing, or modeling, or describing a brain state. But the brain state in question is highly specific. It is not an emotion, or a thought, or a motive. It is attention. In the present theory, the brain constructs a descriptive model of attention. Attention can be applied to a color, a sound, a touch, an emotion, a thought, a movement plan, and many other things external and internal. Attention is not limited to self-attention. It is a general operation that can be applied to almost any type of information. In the present theory, since awareness is a descriptive model of attention, and since attention can be applied to a vast range of information, awareness can encompass the same huge range of information. The theory is not limited to self-knowledge, to a narrative about personal choices, or to any single aspect of mental life. The theory adequately covers the necessary range of information. If the brain can focus attention on X, then according to the present theory, it can be aware of X, because awareness is a model of the act of attention.

Few previous theories of consciousness have this advantage. They apply to some limited set of information, such as self-knowledge, visual information, or information about one's own physical body, and leave unexplained the majority of stuff that can enter awareness. The attention schema theory has the advantage of encompassing the right range of information. If you can pay attention to X, then you can be aware of it.

Consciousness in the Absence of Other People

Another common criticism of the social approach to consciousness is easily explained and easily dismissed. If my consciousness depends on the machinery in my brain for social interaction, and if I am alone, interacting with no other person, then why am I still conscious? How am I aware of the picture on the wall if nobody else is in the room also looking at the same picture? Shouldn't consciousness disappear as soon as I absent myself from a social context?

This common criticism is, to some extent, artificial. Of course, the machinery for social cognition is still present in my brain, whether I am in a social group or not. Even if I were in solitary confinement in jail for a month, my brain would still contain that circuitry, and I could still use that circuitry to construct a narrative or an understanding of myself. To make the point even more obvious with an analogy, the foot evolved mainly for walking. But when I'm not walking, I still have a foot. I don't exactly lose it by virtue of sitting down. I can still use it for tapping a rhythm. Likewise, the machinery in my brain for understanding minds is present and remains present whether I'm at a party, sitting alone in my office, or languishing in solitary confinement. That brain machinery is always there and can always be used to construct an understanding of my own mind.

Why Are Autistic People Conscious?

Social theories of consciousness inevitably encounter a particular challenge. If consciousness is a result of social intelligence, then people with impaired social intelligence should have impaired consciousness. The most thoroughly studied impairment in social capability is autism.[14,15] At the extreme end, people with severe autism can fail to develop any normal social ability, including language. At the more subtle end of the spectrum, people with a high-functioning Asperger's syndrome have some difficulty reading the thoughts and emotions of others. Their condition is more of a personality type than a disorder. Are people on the autistic spectrum less conscious in any way?

The question is difficult to approach, for ethical reasons. To claim that autistic children are less conscious than normal children smacks of dehumanizing the group. Moreover, it is not clear how to measure level of consciousness, especially in a severely autistic child who doesn't talk or engage with other people. How would anyone know? Compounding the problem, especially if the attention schema theory is correct, we humans have a built-in tendency to attribute consciousness to others. Even supposing an autistic person were somehow less conscious than normal, even if that were true, if you spend enough time with that person, you are likely to develop a strong impression of consciousness in that person. You would easily convince yourself that the person was conscious, regardless of the truth of the matter.

At least one study suggests that autistic people are less aware of their own emotions.[16] But autistic people are not necessarily less aware all around. Perhaps autism affects a person's ability to understand emotions. Awareness of the visual world, of auditory experience, of touch and smell seems unimpaired as far as anyone knows, though such things are difficult to measure. The evidence, such as it is, does not obviously support the social theories of consciousness, which predict that autistic people should be all around less aware.

Autism is only one specific example. If consciousness is a construct of the social machinery, then social disabilities and awareness disabilities should correlate. Yet the classical syndromes of social impairment, including autism, social anxiety disorder, schizoid personality disorder, and a sociopathic personality type, are not generally associated with a derangement of conscious experience. At least, that symptom is not emphasized in the classical descriptions.

People who live in forced isolation, Robinson Crusoe style, and who therefore don't practice their social skills show no particular evidence of losing the capacity for conscious experience. People are sometimes born and raised in almost complete social isolation.[17-20] When rescued and studied, such people may show severe disabilities in language and social interaction, but I am not aware of any reports of a general loss of sentience in these cases. If social impairments are associated with a general impairment of consciousness, the relationship is evidently a weak one. There may be a relationship (the question is largely unexplored and is hard to test anyway), but since it has gone unnoticed, it is evidently not black and white or absolute. Since socially impaired people appear to be conscious and can report that they are conscious in much the same way that anyone else does, the evidence is against the theory that social capacity is the source of consciousness.

The fundamental difficulty here is that the social theories of consciousness are too general. They imply that awareness arises from any and all social thinking. They predict a sweeping correlation between all social ability and awareness. The attention schema theory of consciousness avoids this difficulty because it does not suffer from overgenerality. It is much more specific. In it, awareness depends on one specific function, an ability to reconstruct, describe, or model the process of attention. It is not the "social schema" theory but specifically the "attention schema" theory.

A person could be socially impaired in half a dozen ways and have no loss of awareness. A difficulty in recognizing faces, in reading people's expressions, in judging emotions, in reconstructing someone else's thoughts or beliefs, in empathy, in following social norms, in feeling comfortable in a crowd—none of these difficulties should have any particular relationship to a reduction in awareness. In the attention schema theory, there is no reason to suppose that autistic people, or schizoid people, or shy people, or Robinson Crusoe people, or psychopathic malefactors, or any other people with social disabilities are any less conscious than the rest of us. In the attention schema theory, it is at least theoretically possible to have a perfectly functioning attention schema applied to yourself, constructing the feature of awareness and attributing it to yourself, while at the same time, due to a disruption in other aspects of social thinking, be totally unable to attribute awareness to anyone else. You might have no social capacity at all and sit in a huddle walled in your own mental world, and you might never look at anyone else or say a word to anyone else, and yet you would still qualify as conscious in the present theory. In this theory, awareness and social perception are related but not equated. Damage to the attention schema should disrupt one's own awareness and disrupt a specific part of social intelligence, the ability to track or understand other people's attention.

The Knower and the Known

The social theories of consciousness have sometimes been criticized for confusing the knower with the known. They deal in the self-narrative, the information that you think you know about your-self, but they do not explain who the "you" is who knows it. How do you become aware of the information?

In an intuitive view of consciousness, a distinction is made between the information processed in the brain (the known) and the awareness itself (the knower). The two are not considered to be the same type of stuff, however close their relationship may be. Any description of information in the brain addresses Chalmers's easy problem,[21] describing the stuff of which you are aware without addressing the hard problem of how you got to be aware of it.

Social theories of consciousness suffer from precisely this failing. In these theories, the brain constructs information about the self. Your brain invents a narrative in which you are feeling this emotion, your reasons are that, your beliefs are the other. But how do you become aware of that information? Granted that you develop narratives to explain your own behavior, how do you become aware of the information contained in those narratives?

I believe that most scholars have a deep-seated bias in the way they think about consciousness. The bias is pervasive and subtle. In it, awareness and information are distinct from each other. Awareness might be an emanation from information, or a special state of infor-mation, or an operation performed on information, or a thing that receives information like a receptacle. When a metal burner on a stove becomes hot, the heat is an emanation from the metal or, more accu-rately, a state of motion of the metal atoms that can be transmitted to other atoms. The heat is obviously not itself made out of metal. When you cut a banana with a knife, the knife operates on the banana. It makes no sense to postulate that the knife is made out of a banana. A strongbox is something in which treasure can be stored. The strong-box is not itself made out of treasure. Similarly, when you become aware of information in the brain, it is because awareness is a heat-like emanation from information, or a knife-like operation that acts on information, or a receptacle that takes in information. It makes no sense to postulate that awareness itself is made out of information.

This alternative point of view is a true antithesis to the present theory. On the one side lies intuition: awareness can't *be* information, because we become aware *of* information. On the other side lie objectivity and inference: the only thing we know about awareness for certain is that we can at least sometimes decide that we have it and report that we have it. Only information can provide grist to the machinery of decision-making and reporting. Therefore, logically, awareness is information.

How should we resolve this dilemma?

Or, to frame the question differently: suppose for the moment that I am right. Suppose that awareness is information, as I am suggesting. Then why do we have such a strong introspective intuition to the contrary? Why do we find it so natural, so obvious, that awareness operates *on* information and therefore can't itself *be* information?

The attention schema theory provides a neat explanation. The brain contains the process of attention. Attention is a data-handling method. Attention actually does operate on information; it enhances some informational representations in the brain while inhibiting others. Attention actually is an emergent property; it emerges from the competition among signals in the brain. Attention is a state into which information can enter; select information gets into the focus of attention. Attention is not itself information. It is something that *happens to* information. Attention may be a mechanistic process, it may be something programmable into a computer, but its relationship to information is suspiciously like the intuitive relationship between awareness and information.

In the present theory, the brain constructs an informational model to usefully represent the process of attention. By introspecting, by accessing that model and examining its properties, we cannot escape the intuition that we become aware *of* information, that awareness emerges *from* information, that awareness operates *on* information, or that awareness is a state into which information enters. The informational model depicts those particular properties because it is depicting attention and attention actually has those properties.

Cart and Horse: Which Came First, Personal Consciousness or Attributing Consciousness to Someone Else?

Social theories of consciousness are sometimes criticized for putting the cart before the horse. In the social theories of consciousness, humans developed an ability to understand other people's minds. Once having gained that special machinery, we then evolved or learned the ability to turn it on ourselves, and in that way gained self-understanding. This order of development seems backward to some thinkers. A more common intuition is that we understand ourselves first, and with that self-familiarity as a basis we use empathy to understand others. We somehow have an ability to "see" inside our own minds and directly experience our own emotions, thoughts, and sensory impressions. Given this ability, we are able to understand other people by imagining ourselves in their shoes. In this more common view, self-knowledge precedes knowledge of others. Consciousness precedes social perception.

Which came first, the ability to understand other people's minds, or the ability to understand one's own mind?

The attention schema theory is agnostic on the question of which came first. It escapes any horse-and-cart issue entirely. The question remains open: in evolution, did we develop our own awareness first, or did we attribute awareness to other people first? Consider the evolutionary possibilities.

Possibility 1: Awareness of Self Came First and Attributing Awareness to Others Followed

Modeling one's own attention is of great use in predicting one's own behavior. Predicting one's own behavior is of great use in planning one's own actions. Therefore (in Possibility 1), the brain evolved a mechanism for modeling its attentional state. Once such a mechanism existed, it could be elaborated and extended to other uses. For example, modeling one's own attention is merely the beginning of building a complex model of one's mind state in general. Constructing a model of one's own mind state can be adapted to the task of modeling the mind states of others. In this way a possible evolutionary path can be traced, from the simpler initial task of monitoring one's own attention ultimately to the vastly more elaborated task, greatly expanded in humans, of social intelligence.

Consciousness first; social perception second.

In this speculation, awareness, a continuous model of one's own attentional state, is evolutionarily old, existing in at least some simple form in almost all animals with brains, as long as they have brains capable of the process of attention. If a brain can use attention to sort its signals and shape its behavior, then it can usefully model attention to better understand and predict its own behavior; thus awareness, or the attention schema, becomes an adaptive trait. In contrast, a high level of social intelligence is a recent evolutionary product elaborated mainly in a few mammalian and avian species. Consciousness must be widespread in the animal kingdom, even though social capability is not.

Possibility 2: Attributing Awareness to Others Came First and Personal Awareness Followed

The cerebral cortex of monkeys contains a set of brain areas, a processing stream, that uses visual information to recognize objects.[22] In this processing stream, each successive brain region is better able to extract information such as color, shape, texture, and ultimately the identity of an object. At the highest levels of this processing stream, neurons respond to socially relevant cues, including visual images of faces, gaze direction, and body gestures.[23-29]

These findings on the visual system suggest, at least as a speculation, that animals first evolved the ability to process sensory information. They then evolved a special ability to process the nuanced, complex sensory information that indicates the behavior of other animals. From there the machinery evolved to compute inferences about the mental states of other animals. Once the circuitry was capable of attributing mental states to others, it could then be used to attribute mental states to oneself, leading to consciousness. In this account, social perception evolved over a long span of time as an outgrowth of sensory processing, but consciousness arose quite recently in evolution.

I do not know which of these two evolutionary possibilities is correct. Perhaps awareness is evolutionarily old and is widespread in the animal kingdom. Perhaps it is new and is limited to a few, highly social and intelligent species. Perhaps both evolutionary paths contributed and different aspects of consciousness emerged gradually at different times. (That combination is my current best guess.) My reason for explicitly laying out the alternate possibilities is to make the point that they are all compatible with the present theory. There is no cart-and-horse difficulty here. Whichever came first, whether attributing consciousness to oneself or to others, the attention schema theory remains unchallenged by this particular issue. Only more data will enable us to determine whether something like an attention schema exists at all, whether it exists in a range of animals, or whether it is limited to those with an elaborated social processing machinery.

Improving on the Social Theories of Consciousness

In this chapter I described a common, recurring hypothesis: consciousness is the result of social intelligence, our ability to understand the minds of other people, turned inward on ourselves. That general approach has many variants but they all involve a core idea: we invent a plausible, after-the-fact story to account for our actions, just as we do to account for the actions of the people around us.

The general hypothesis has some validity to it. But this type of theory does a poor job of explaining consciousness. It explains a type of knowledge while saying nothing about awareness itself. It is limited to self-knowledge and says nothing about knowledge of external information such as color or sound. It fails to explain why socially impaired people, such as autistic people, are apparently just as aware as the rest of us. Pet owners should be skeptical of the social approach to consciousness. It implies that pets and other animals with limited social cognition are not truly conscious.

The theory proposed in this book, the attention schema theory, is related to the social theories of consciousness. Yet the attention schema theory avoids the standard pitfalls. Its strength lies in its specificity. It is not a theory that equates any and all social capacity with one's own private awareness. Instead, the theory focuses on one attribute: how do we understand that person Y is attending to thing X? How do we understand the attentional state of another person? How do we understand our own attentional state? The theory posits a specific construct, a model or a schema that is constantly updated and recomputed, a chunk of information that represents attention. Awareness is that attention schema.

The theory is not merely about self-knowledge but about awareness itself. It is about the knower, not just the known. It explains why we attribute a particular, quirky set of properties to awareness. It accounts for awareness in all the right domains, such as vision, touch, emotion, ideas, and memories. It accounts for both self-awareness and awareness of the external world. It allows for awareness in people who might be socially challenged.

If the attention schema theory were solely a tweak or refinement of the social theories of consciousness, avoiding some of the typical pitfalls of that common previous approach, it would probably still deserve consideration. The theory, however, has a much broader scope. The next six chapters, most of the rest of this book, take up a great range of topics in consciousness research and in brain research. These topics include previous theories of how the brain produces consciousness, how social intelligence is organized in the brain, how damage to the brain may disrupt consciousness, how specific neurons in the brain may help mirror the thoughts and actions of others, and many other subjects. All of these topics relate in a fundamental way to the attention schema theory. The theory may be able to pull together a large set of otherwise disparate findings and hypotheses into a single framework.

11

Consciousness as Integrated Information

In the previous chapter I discussed one of the most common theoretical approaches to consciousness—the social construction of consciousness. A second common theoretical approach is to attribute consciousness to informational complexity and in particular to the linking, or binding, or integration of information in the brain. The social approach and the integrated information approach to consciousness are quite different and in some ways have been viewed as rivals. Yet the attention schema theory could be seen as a way of fusing the two approaches.

In the attention schema theory, awareness is a computed feature. It is descriptive information—call it information set A. To be aware of X is to bind or integrate the information that depicts X with the information set A. When you report that you are aware of X, it is because cognitive machinery in your brain has accessed that large, brain-spanning set of information, $A + X$, and is summarizing it. You are reporting that X comes with the properties of A attached to it. The attention schema theory works only so far as the proposed attention schema can be bound to other chunks of information. It is an integrated information approach to consciousness just as much as it is a social approach.

This chapter describes the integrated information approach to consciousness, beginning with the early versions of that line of thinking, and then discussing some of the potential strengths and weaknesses of the approach and how it may relate specifically to the attention schema theory.

Integrated Information Theories

In 1983, Baars[1,2] proposed the global workspace hypothesis, one of the first well-articulated theories of consciousness as integrated information. In that theory, information spanning many brain areas can be linked or bound into a single, coherent whole, and that brain-wide pool of information forms a global workspace that encompasses the contents of consciousness.

The neural basis for binding information across widespread brain areas is not yet known, but one hypothesis has been investigated in some depth. In 1990, Singer and colleagues[3] were studying the visual system of the cat and discovered that under some conditions the neurons were active in rhythmic bursts. These bursts occurred about 40 times per second in a regular oscillation. Moreover, different neurons that were spatially separated from each other in the cortex could oscillate in synchrony with each other.

In theory, two neurons that are active in synchrony form a powerful information unit. A single neuron, sending a signal, may fail to impact the downstream circuitry, or impact it in a marginal way that does not rise above the level of random fluctuation. But two or more neurons firing in synchrony, sending their signals to the same downstream collector, can have a coherent impact that rises above the background noise. Singer and colleagues proposed that the synchronization of neurons was a means of binding together the information carried by those neurons into a single informational unit. When one neuron caries information A, and another neuron carries information B, and those two neurons are active in synchrony, then information A has been linked with or bound to information B, the two chunks of information passed to downstream circuitry as $A + B$. That, at least, is the essence of the hypothesis.

Synchrony and oscillations have since been found in the cat, monkey, mouse, rat, and human, and the synchrony does indeed increase in situations when the brain binds many different pieces of information into a perceptual whole.[4]

Recent work on oscillations in the monkey and human cortex suggests that periods of oscillation can open up between two distant regions of the cortex.[5-7] As the two cortical areas are active in synchronized oscillations, they become better able to transmit information from one to the other. The period of oscillation acts like a portal for efficient information transfer.

Shortly after cortical oscillations were first discovered, in 1990, Crick and Koch[8] proposed one of the first mechanistic, neuronal theories of consciousness. They suggested that consciousness was linked to the synchronized neuronal activity that may bind information together across the brain. In their theory, consciousness arises as a result of complex, bound information that can be maintained over long enough intervals to enter short-term memory.

Many scientists have since reiterated and emphasized the same general hypothesis: consciousness occurs when information is bound into complex units that span many disparate brain regions.[2,4,6,9-13]

A recent theory of this type, in which consciousness is a complex, bound set of information, was proposed by Tononi.[14,15] In Tononi's integrated information hypothesis, as information becomes linked in increasingly complex ways, consciousness emerges. He describes the example of looking at a white screen. A simple machine equipped with a photodiode can register the information that the screen is bright. But the machine presumably has no conscious experience of whiteness. Why? In Tononi's account, it is because the machine encodes impoverished information. A human has a vast linked set of visual information, including the luminance of the screen; the whiteness of the screen; the distinction between white and the many colors that are not present on the screen, between white and black, between white and red, between white and any other location in the vast informational space of the color wheel; information about the texture of the screen, about the borders of the screen, and so on. The sheer immensity of information encoded in the person's brain about a white screen is starkly different from the simple, low-bit information of the machine with the photodiode. In Tononi's hypothesis, this informational complexity in the human brain is why the human has a conscious experience and the machine does not. In that hypothesis, the conscious experience of whiteness is tantamount to the vast network of bound information in the human brain that is invoked by looking at the white screen. Consciousness is integrated information. As the amount of integrated information increases, consciousness emerges. As the integrated information is reduced, consciousness should fade.

Tononi's hypothesis is stripped of reference to the neuronal underpinning. Whether synchronous neuronal activity truly provides the mechanism is irrelevant to the deeper concept. Let the hardware be what it is, the essence of the theory is that information, bound in a rich enough interconnected network, becomes conscious.

In the following sections I outline three potential difficulties with the integrated information theory and discuss how these difficulties might be resolved by the attention schema theory. My goal here is not to argue against the integrated information approach. I am not trying to knock it down and set up a new theory. On the contrary, I argue that the approach is valuable, and that some nagging problems with it disappear when it is considered from a new perspective and combined with ideas from a different source.

Integrated Information Is Not Always Conscious

Most processing systems in the brain have no relationship to consciousness.

For example, we move fluidly, easily, coordinating hundreds of muscles, forces, joint angles, and joint speeds, without any consciousness of exactly how. The computations that guide the intercoordinated nuance of muscle control are outside of awareness. Only very general aspects of movement control and movement goals ever reach consciousness. The highly integrated computations that control heart rate, blood vessel constriction, hormonal content, digestive activity, temperature, and other matters of the inner environment, occur outside of awareness.

A part of the human cerebral cortex, the posterior parietal lobe, appears to play a special role in hand–eye coordination. Goodale and colleagues proposed that this brain area functions largely outside of consciousness.[16,17] They studied a patient who, due to diffuse brain damage, no longer had any awareness of the shapes, sizes, or orientations of objects in front of her. Despite the brain damage, the patient still had intact parietal lobes. If asked to reach out and grasp an object, the patient would confidently do so, with the correct hand orientation and the correct finger shaping, even though she insisted she was not conscious of the shape or location of the object. When asked to post a letter in a slot, the patient could do so easily, despite having no awareness of the shape of the letter or the orientation of the slot. In contrast, people who had damage to the parietal lobe suffered the opposite set of difficulties. They were unable to reach, grasp, or manipulate objects. They reached to the wrong places, grasped the wrong parts of the objects, and opened their fingers to the wrong extent. Yet they reported a perfect awareness of the objects in front of them, including shapes and sizes. Goodale concluded that the parietal lobe was critical for hand–eye coordination but did not contribute to conscious experience. That brain region carried out its computations outside of consciousness. Yet the parietal lobe contains information as intensively integrated as in any other region of the brain. Indeed, the parietal cortex is one of the main integrative hubs in the brain.

People can be primed to perform complex tasks without even knowing they are doing so. These tasks can include decoding the emotions in a face, recognizing the identity of a face, registering the meaning of words, registering the mathematical meaning of numbers, and other astonishing feats of perception and cognition occurring under the surface of consciousness.[18] For example, if the word *frog* is flashed on a screen in front of you—if it is flashed quickly—you will have no awareness of the word. You might report seeing a flash of light, but no letters. Yet if after that you are asked for a word that begins with *f*, any word—just blurt out the first word that comes to mind—you are more likely to say "frog" than would be expected by chance. Something in your bran must have processed the word. These tasks require the integration of information, yet can be done without awareness.

Brain systems that operate outside of awareness have been called "zombie units."[19] Proponents of the integrated information theory might suggest that the zombie units are unconscious because the information in them is less integrated. For my own tastes, however, this explanation seems too convenient. It is too easy to look at a system that does not contribute to consciousness and find, with a little effort, a reason to convince oneself that its information is less integrated. It is too easy to look at a system that participates in consciousness and, again with a little effort, convince oneself that its information is more integrated. When you coordinate your hand and eye, blending the visual input and the muscle control, most of that coordination is computed outside of awareness. But I have a hard time believing that the relevant information is in any way lacking integration. My background in neuroscience lies in the control of movement, so I have an appreciation for the incredible amount of information that needs to be integrated to make any kind of coordinated movement possible.

Computer technology has reached a point where vast, interconnected networks of information are now possible. The Internet, as far as anyone can tell, is not conscious. Deep Blue, the IBM chess machine, shows no signs of consciousness. Neither does Watson, the machine that plays Jeopardy. A giant interlinked tax code is not conscious. (At least I hope not.)

To save the integrated information hypothesis of consciousness, one could argue that these complex, information-processing entities are actually conscious but simply don't have the verbal skills to say so. Maybe the computer on your desk is aware of itself but lacks the ability to communicate that state. This type of argument, however, weakens rather than strengthens the integrated information theory. It is a poor argument to point to something for which there is no evidence of any consciousness and then claim that it is conscious but just can't say so. The argument is vacuous because it has no limits and can be applied to anything. Maybe rocks are conscious but just can't say so. It is a variant on, "You have no evidence against it, so it must be true," a thoroughly antiscientific argument.

The underlying difficulty here is that integrated information is ubiquitous. Therefore, a theory that equates consciousness with integrated information is left trying to explain why so much integrated information in the world, including much of it in our heads, shows no signs of consciousness.

The attention schema theory does not suffer from this difficulty of overgenerality. In this theory, consciousness is not the result of integrated information in general. It depends instead on a specific kind of information. It is not a theory in which one's cell phone, having become sufficiently integrated with other cell phones, experiences consciousness.

According to the attention schema theory, the brain constructs a constantly shifting, constantly updated informational model or schema, A. The schema provides a depiction of what it means for a brain to deeply process, apprehend, attend to, and *seize* information. This schema can be bound to other informational representations in the brain. To be conscious of a visual stimulus, in this formulation, at minimum a bound representation $A + V$ is required, where V stands for the information about the visual stimulus, presumably represented in visual circuitry. With this larger, integrated information set, the brain has the basis for concluding and reporting that V is present and that V comes attached to the properties described in A. In other words, the brain has the basis for concluding that the visual stimulus comes with an inner conscious experience.

To know that you, your own physical and mental self, are aware of a visual stimulus requires, by hypothesis, the larger bound representation $S + A + V$. Here S refers to the complex, vast information set that defines your understanding of yourself. The larger, integrated complex of information provides the basis for a brain to conclude that V is present, that it comes with an inner experience, and that you, in particular, are the one experiencing it.

To be conscious of your own emotions requires a bound representation $S + A + E$, where E stands for the information about emotional state.

To be conscious that you are doing mental arithmetic requires the bound representation $S + A + M$, where M stands for the computed mathematical information.

In the present theory, only information bound to the attention schema is recognized or describable as being within consciousness. The attention schema, A, acts like a hub. It is the nexus at the center of a vast set of bound information, represented in diverse brain areas, that makes up the contents of consciousness.

Because of this involvement of a large bound set of information that spans the brain, the attention schema theory is a type of integrated information theory. It shares similarities with Baars's global workspace hypothesis,[1,2] with Crick and Koch's theory of binding as the basis of consciousness,[8] and with Tononi's integrated information theory.[14] But it does not suffer from the problem of overgenerality. It is not enough to pool information into a global workspace. It is not enough to accumulate a large pile of interlinked information. In the attention schema theory, what people call "awareness" depends on a specific set of information integrated into that global workspace. Awareness itself, in this theory, is a complex, continuously recomputed model that describes what it means—the conditions, dynamics, and consequences—for a brain to attentively process information. When that information is added to the mix, the system has a basis on which to decide that it is conscious, report that it is conscious, and describe some of the attributes of consciousness. Without that information, the system logically has no way to compute what consciousness is or whether it has it. The system can admirably compute other types of information—visual information, tactile information, mental arithmetic—and answer questions thereof. But lacking the relevant information set, it would be silent both inwardly and outwardly on the topic of consciousness.

In the present theory, consciousness is not integrated information per se. Rather, we are conscious of information that is integrated with an attention schema.

The Difficulties of Testing the Integrated Information Theory

How can the integrated information theory of consciousness be tested? Theoretically, there are two approaches. First, one could try to create consciousness artificially by building an integrated set of information. Second, one could try to remove consciousness from something that already has it by de-integrating the information.

The first approach would be to build a system that includes integrated information and then to speculate about whether the system is conscious. The difficulty, as noted in the previous section, is that the claim of consciousness is unverifiable. You could build a computer, put in a good dose of integrated information, and then boldly claim that the computer is conscious. Alas, the computer lacks the verbal skills to say so, and so the test is less than useful.

The second approach would be to test whether human consciousness fades when integration in the brain is reduced. Tononi[17] emphasizes the case of anesthesia. As a person is anesthetized, integration among the many parts of the brain slowly decreases, and so does consciousness. Someone naïve to the dangers of correlation might mistake this finding as support for the theory. But even without doing the experiment, we already know what the result must be. As the brain degrades in its function, so does the integration among its various parts and so does the intensity of awareness. But so do most other functions. Even many unconscious processes in the brain depend on integration of information and will degrade as integration deteriorates.

The underlying difficulty here is once again the generality of integrated information. Integrated information is so pervasive and so necessary for almost all complex functions in the brain that the theory is essentially unfalsifiable. Whatever consciousness may be, it depends in some manner on integrated information and decreases as integration in the brain is compromised.

The attention schema theory has the advantage of greater specificity. Not any integrated information gives rise to consciousness, only the attention schema integrated with other pieces of information. Find the system in the human brain that computes the attention schema, and the theory is directly testable. Knock out that system, and awareness should disappear. Damage part of that system, and awareness should be severely compromised. Alter the processing in that system, and the nature of consciousness should be warped. Where this system might be located in the brain, and what happens when those brain areas are disrupted, is discussed in later chapters.

Explaining the Reportability of Consciousness

The only objective, physically measurable truth we have about consciousness is that we can, at least sometimes, report that we have it. I can say, "The apple is green," like a well-regulated wavelength detector, providing no evidence of consciousness; but I can also claim, "I am sentient; I have a conscious experience of green."

One of the advantages of the social theories of consciousness, whatever their weaknesses may be, is that they explain the reportability of consciousness. Indeed, they are *about* the reportability of consciousness. In that approach, consciousness is a narrative that the brain constructs to explain itself. Gazzaniga's interpreter, for example, is a language-talented left hemisphere reporting on its motives at least as it has reconstructed them.

The attention schema theory has the same advantage. It explains the reportability of consciousness. We can report that we have awareness because it is a schema, a complex set of information that can be cognitively accessed and from which summaries can be abstracted and verbalized. We can report that we have experiences because the having of an experience is depicted in the information set.

Many previous approaches to consciousness do not address the question of reportability. The integrated information view belongs to this category. It is silent on how we get from being conscious to being able to report, "I have a conscious experience." Yet any serious theory of consciousness must explain the one objective fact that we have about consciousness: that we can, in principle, at least sometimes, report that we have it.

In discussion with colleagues, I have heard the following argument that I think may capture a deep and unspoken assumption. The brain has highly integrated information. Highly integrated information is (so the theory goes) consciousness. Problem solved. Why do we need a special mechanism to inform the brain about something that it already has? The integrated information is already in there; therefore, the brain should be able to report that it has it.

When put explicitly, this argument has some obvious gaps. The brain contains a lot of items that it can't report. The brain contains synapses, but nobody can introspect and say, "Yup, those serotonin synapses are particularly itchy today." The brain regulates the flow of blood through itself, but nobody has cognitive access to that process either. For a brain to be able to report on something, the relevant item can't merely be present in the brain but must be encoded as information in the form of neural signals that can ultimately inform the speech circuitry.

The integrated information theory of consciousness does not explain how the brain, possessing integrated information (and, therefore, by hypothesis consciousness), encodes the fact that it has consciousness, so that consciousness can be explicitly acknowledged and reported. One would be able to report, "The apple is green," like a well-calibrated spectral analysis machine. One would be able to report, "The green here is darker; the green there is lighter; the green is not white; the green is not red; the skin of the apple provides a shiny texture; there is a bright reflection here but not there; the apple is almost round but dented at the top." One would be able to report a great range of information that is indeed integrated. The information is all of a type that a sophisticated visual processing computer, attached to a camera, could decode and report. But there is no proposed mechanism for the brain to arrive at the conclusion, "Hey, green is a conscious *experience*." How does the presence of conscious experience get turned into a report?

To get around this difficulty and save the integrated information theory, we would have to postulate that the integrated information that makes up consciousness includes not just information that depicts the apple but also information that depicts what a conscious experience is, what awareness itself is, what it means to experience. The two chunks of information would need to be linked. Then the system would be able to report that it has a conscious experience of the apple. In that case, the integrated information theory and the attention schema theory converge and become the same theory. I suggest this is the correct way to modify the integrated information approach to resolve its difficulties.

Toward the beginning of this book, in Chapter 2, I described a schematic formulation of the problem of consciousness (see Figure 2.2), Arrow A is the mysterious process by which neuronal machinery leads to consciousness. Arrow B is the mysterious process by which consciousness causes changes in neuronal machinery, allowing us to report that we have it. Almost all theories of consciousness address themselves to Arrow A and ignore the presence of Arrow B. But Arrow B is the only scientific handle that we have on consciousness. The fact that consciousness can at least sometimes be reported is its only verifiable attribute. Any scientific theory of consciousness must explain in principle how the stuff can lead to our ability to report its presence. The attention schema theory is, in its essence, the result of working backward from the reportability of consciousness while keeping within the constraints of the brain as an information-processing device.

12

Neural Correlates of Consciousness

In the last two chapters I discussed some prominent scientific theories of consciousness that fell into two general categories: the social perception approach and the integrated information approach. Not all scientific work on consciousness, however, is driven by theory. One useful approach to consciousness is more look-and-see: study the brain itself, examine any quirks of perception or quirks of brain function that might be relevant to the question, and keep one's scientific eyes open in case insight can be gained.

The difficulty with this explorative approach, however, is that one must look in the right place. It is difficult to guide the exploration without a theory to point the way. In my view, the experimental search has generally been directed to the wrong places in the brain.

This explorative, experimental approach has tended to focus mostly on visual awareness. How does the brain become conscious of a visual image? To find the neuronal substrate of visual awareness, scientists tend to look to visual circuitry. That is where visual information is processed, and therefore (in the common view at least) that ought to be the site from which the awareness of visual information emerges. By analogy, tactile awareness must emerge from somatosensory circuitry. Emotional awareness must emerge from those brain regions that compute emotions. Awareness of mental arithmetic must emerge from whatever brain circuitry performs the computations of mental arithmetic. In this common view, the brain must generate consciousness from many places simultaneously like steam rising here and there from leaky pipes. In such a view, it is not absolutely clear why some brain systems generate consciousness and others do not. It is also not clear how all these disparate sources of consciousness can result in what seems, introspectively, to be a unified consciousness. It is even less clear how the property of consciousness, once generated in one place in the brain, such as in visual cortex, can be transmitted to a different site in the brain, such that it can join with other instances of consciousness or flow into and affect speech circuitry. Is consciousness transmitted along neuronal fibers, the same way that regular information is transmitted? If so, then what exactly is the difference between consciousness and information? These issues have remained somewhat obscure.

In the attention schema theory, consciousness does not, so to speak, *emerge* from information, but instead it *is* information. It is information of a specific type. It is information that describes the process of attending to something. In the case of visual consciousness, the brain binds together information about the visual image that is being attended (V), information about the agent performing the attention (S), and a schema, or information structure, that roughly represents the dynamics and implications of attention (A). A brain-spanning representation is formed, $S + A + V$. We can report that we have visual consciousness because the cognitive machinery can read that representation and summarize what is described by it. If this theory is correct, then visual circuitry by itself will not provide the answer to visual consciousness. Something else is computing the consciousness part of visual consciousness, the awareness, the A part of $S + A + V$.

The search for the brain basis of consciousness has tended to target sensory areas where, according to the attention schema theory, the answer is not to be found. Perhaps for this reason, this experimental approach has not fared well. It has certainly failed to uncover a coherent explanation of consciousness. The experiments and observations are nonetheless interesting and important. The attention schema theory, if it is correct, had better be consistent with these experimental observations.

The following sections briefly summarize two common experimental approaches to the neuronal correlates of consciousness. These studies look for events in the brain that correlate with the presence or absence of visual consciousness.

Binocular Rivalry

One popular experimental paradigm for studying consciousness involves a visual trick called binocular rivalry.[1-3] In binocular rivalry, two different images are presented simultaneously, one to each eye. People report that they consciously see one or the other image, almost never both. The percept switches from image to image somewhat unpredictably every few seconds in what is called a bistable fashion. If you have an image of Dorothy presented to one eye and the Wicked Witch of the West to the other eye, you will see Dorothy; a moment later she will fade and give rise to the wicked witch; and in another moment, the witch will fade and cede the visual field once again to Dorothy.

The logic goes as follows: if you can find the consciousness part of the brain, then neurons in that brain area should change their activity levels every few seconds, tracking the image that is currently in consciousness. When the person is aware of Dorothy, neurons in that brain area should respond as though only Dorothy were present. When the person is aware of the witch, the neurons should respond as though only the witch were present. For example, a neuron that codes for green, if it is in a consciousness area of the brain, should be active only when the wicked witch with her green skin rises into consciousness. In contrast, a visual brain area that does not participate in consciousness, that merely processes whatever comes in through the eyes, should be active in the same, unchanging pattern, regardless of whether Dorothy or the witch has risen into consciousness, because the actual visual stimulation to the eyes is constant.

If anyone hoped to find a specific visual-consciousness network using this method, the hope was disappointed. The answer seemed to be smeared out over the entire visual system.[1,3,4] No specific network of brain areas stood out as the site of visual consciousness. Some evidence of an effect of binocular rivalry was found almost everywhere, with more of an effect in areas that were higher up the processing hierarchy.

In the end, the lessons about consciousness from binocular rivalry are ambiguous. A major part of the ambiguity comes from the correlational nature of the experiment. Even if a particular brain area responds in a manner correlated with visual consciousness, do those neurons necessarily cause consciousness? Perhaps they pipe information to some other part of the brain that constructs consciousness. Or perhaps the critical information flows back to those visual neurons. Perhaps some other relationship exists between consciousness and the responses of those particular neurons. The experiment is correlational, with all the interpretational difficulties of that type of study. Correlation does not imply causation.

At least one clear pattern emerges from the binocular rivalry literature. When one visual stimulus rises into consciousness, its signals throughout the visual cortex grow stronger and more consistent.[1,3–5] This finding probably fits with most theories of consciousness. It is certainly consistent with the attention schema theory. In the attention schema theory, visual information encoded in visual cortex will join reportable consciousness only when it is strong enough, or consistent enough, or in some other way boosted enough, to robustly impact other brain systems and in that way become linkable to the attention schema.

I do not mean to suggest that the attention schema theory provides a detailed mechanistic explanation of the results from binocular rivalry. The experiments, because of their correlational nature, are open to multiple interpretations. But the results from that body of work are at least consistent with the attention schema theory. Perhaps I should say the results from binocular rivalry are at least not *inconsistent* with the attention schema theory.

Blindsight

One of the best-studied syndromes related to consciousness is blindsight.[6,7] The cerebral cortex contains an area at the back of the brain called the primary visual cortex. Most visual information that gets into the cortex reaches the primary visual cortex first and then is sent on to other cortical regions. When the primary visual cortex is damaged, such as from a stroke, people report that they are blind in the affected part of visual space. Since the primary visual cortex contains a map of visual space, damage to one part of the map will affect visual processing for only one specific region of the visual world. For example, a patient might be blind in the upper right quadrant. The patient reports a total lack of visual conscious experience in the blind region.

If you seat a patient of this type in front of a screen and present visual images in the blind region, the patient denies seeing anything. The patient may even remind you, "I'm blind there. Why even bother asking?" But if pressed to guess, many patients can indicate exactly when the image appears. They can point accurately to the stimulus and can sometimes report about its motion and brightness, all the while insisting that nothing is present and that the answers are random guesses. Clearly visual processing is present, visual information is present, and the ability for that information to guide movement is present. But visual consciousness is not present. The brain processes the information, but the information does not reach awareness. Primary visual cortex seems to be necessary for visual awareness. In blindsight, whatever regions of the brain are still receiving visual input, processing it, and responding to it, they are evidently unable to lead to awareness.

One common interpretation is that primary visual cortex *creates* awareness. Perhaps something in its circuitry, in the way its neurons pass information among each other, or in its chemical composition or electrical oscillations, produces awareness as a side product. Perhaps awareness is an aura that rises up from primary visual cortex.

The attention schema theory provides an alternative explanation. The primary visual cortex does not, itself, create awareness. Instead, visual information that is computed in it and flows from it is necessary, either directly or indirectly via some cortical middleman, for the V part in $S + A + V$. Other brain systems compute the A part and the S part. All of this information must be bound together to form the basis for reportable visual consciousness. In the attention schema theory, disrupting visual cortex may block visual information from reaching awareness, but it does not disrupt the mechanism of awareness itself. One must look elsewhere in the brain to find the mechanism of awareness—to find the attention schema.

Looking Outside Visual Cortex for Visual Awareness

Both blindsight and binocular rivalry are intriguing phenomena. They are clearly related to consciousness and clearly traceable to specific events in the brain. But the research tends to get bogged down when it comes to interpretation. What, specifically, can be inferred about consciousness from the experimental results?

The problem is that the results do not narrow the possibilities very much. They are consistent with a large range of theories. At least the results set some experimental limits. Any plausible theory of consciousness must be consistent with them. My point in this chapter is that the attention schema theory passes this particular test. It is not ruled out by the standard findings on binocular rivalry or on blindsight. The data are at least not inconsistent with the theory.

But we can do better. We do not need to settle for data that are not inconsistent with the theory. We can find more stringent tests. We can look for experimental results that are difficult to explain *except* by invoking the attention schema theory. We can search for patterns in the data that are specifically predicted by the theory.

As I noted at the beginning of this chapter, in my view too much of the work on consciousness has focused on how visual information, processed in visual areas of the brain, might result in visual consciousness. Certainly both the blindsight literature and the binocular rivalry literature fall into this category. Yet if the attention schema theory is correct, then these previous approaches are looking in the wrong parts of the brain. We should look outside the visual system to find brain areas that might compute the attention schema itself, the awareness construct, the A part of $S + A + V$. The next chapter considers whether anything like the attention schema can be found in the neuronal machinery responsible for social perception.

13

Awareness and the Machinery for Social Perception

If the attention schema theory is correct, then at the center of awareness lies a computed and constantly recomputed informational model, the attention schema. In Chapter 7, I discussed some of the evidence that the human brain uses a model of this type, an attention schema, to monitor and predict the behavior of other people. By hypothesis, the brain could use the same machinery to compute a model of its own attentional state, to help predict and guide its own behavior. In that way we attribute awareness to others and to ourselves.

Social neuroscience is the study of the brain systems that help us think about other people. A widespread set of brain areas is recruited when people engage in social perception. These areas participate in modeling the inner mental states of others. But do these areas model, in particular, the shifting state of attention? Are they able to use that model equally for understanding other people and for understanding oneself?

This chapter reviews some basic information on social neuroscience. At the end of the chapter I evaluate whether any of the social brain areas might participate in awareness—not just in attributing awareness to other people, but also in constructing one's own awareness.

Initial Discoveries in Social Neuroscience

Arguably, social neuroscience began with a discovery in the 1960s by Charles Gross and his colleagues.[1,2] They studied visual processing in the monkey brain. They did not set out to study social processing, but monkeys are highly social animals, and in retrospect it is not surprising that socially relevant signals were discovered at the highest levels of the visual system. Gross and colleagues focused their study on a region of the brain called the inferior temporal cortex, shown in Figure 13.1. Neurons in this region became active in response to the sight of objects. A subset of the neurons, about five percent, became active only when the monkey was shown a face—either a real face or a picture of a face. Another subset of neurons responded to the sight of a hand. These stimuli are of obvious social importance to monkeys.

Further work on the monkey brain revealed a second cortical area that seemed to process an even greater range of socially relevant information. This area, the superior temporal polysensory area (STP), is also shown in Figure 13.1. A high percentage of neurons in this area responded when monkeys were shown pictures of faces, pictures of eyes in particular, and movies of bodies and limbs in action.[3–7]

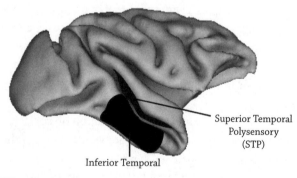

Superior Temporal
Polysensory
(STP)

Inferior Temporal

FIGURE 13.1

Some areas of the monkey brain relevant to social intelligence.

I saw some of the later experiments in Gross's lab on area STP in the monkey brain and witnessed one particularly common class of neuron. "Looming" neurons responded best when a person walked up and loomed toward the monkey's face. Such looming responses were a puzzle at the time, but now I wonder if they might have been related to personal space, another socially relevant property. Area STP seems to be the hot spot in the monkey brain for processing socially relevant signals. It has the highest concentration of such signals, at least that has been found yet.

These remarkable results from the monkey brain were extended to the human brain, mainly by scanning people using an MRI. Kanwisher and colleagues were the first to report a region of the human cortex that responded more strongly to the sight of faces than to other objects.[8]

A fold in the cortex called the superior temporal sulcus (STS) is a particular hotspot of social processing in the human brain. It seems to correspond to the monkey STP both in its functions and its location

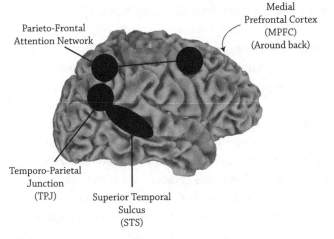

FIGURE 13.2

Some areas of the human brain relevant to social intelligence and to the control of attention.

in the brain. The human STS is shown in Figure 13.2. This cortical area becomes active when a person sees or thinks about the intentional actions of other people, such as hand actions, or changes in gaze direction, or facial expressions.[9-15] It reacts differently to clearly goal-directed actions, such as a movie of a hand reaching out to grasp a cup, than it does to non-goal-directed actions, such as an arm movement that looks as though it has no purpose.[16] Even when a person views simple geometric shapes that move on a computer screen, when the movements are perceived as intentional—the triangle "wanted" to touch that square—then the STS becomes active.[17] The STS therefore may be computing something about the perceived intentions of others.

These many findings suggest that the highest level of the primate visual system, whether in the human or monkey, contains machinery for processing the sensory cues that are most relevant to social interaction.

Brain Areas Recruited During Social Cognition

In social psychology, the concept of social intelligence goes far beyond recognizing other people's faces, monitoring other people's gaze, or noting other people's hand actions. These functions, though important, are arguably basic perceptual building blocks on which a more sophisticated social intelligence must be built. Do any areas or networks in the brain specialize in more complex social cognition?

One aspect of social cognition is termed "theory of mind."[18,19] Theory of mind refers to the ability of a person to construct a model or theory about the contents of someone else's mind. Theory of mind is often tested in a controlled and reduced way by using the "false belief" task.[20] In this task, a person is told a story. Sally and Anne are having a picnic. They've brought two covered baskets. Sally puts a sandwich into basket A and then goes for a walk. While she is gone, Anne sneakily moves the sandwich to basket B. When Sally comes back, which basket will she look in first, to find the sandwich? The correct answer is A. Sally believes the sandwich is in basket A, even though that belief is false. To answer the question correctly, a person must keep track of Sally's beliefs, in effect constructing a model of the contents of Sally's mind.

When people perform this type of task, the false-belief task or other tasks that tap into social cognition, a specific network of cortical areas tends to be recruited. Many of the same brain areas show up regularly in a great range of experiments. Three areas in particular are most commonly reported.[21-28] These areas are shown in Figure 13.2. They include the superior temporal sulcus (STS), the temporo-parietal junction (TPJ), and the medial prefrontal cortex (MPFC). The STS and the TPJ are adjacent to each other and in some ways could be considered part of a larger cortical region that may have distinct subregions. The MPFC is separated from the others. It lies in the frontal lobe and near the midline of the brain. Each area is doubled—one in the right hemisphere, one in the left—but the activity during social cognition is almost always much stronger in the right hemisphere. Other brain areas are also active during social cognition, but the three noted here are among the most commonly studied.

The findings summarized in this section imply that a distinct set of cortical areas is dedicated to social processing. This interpretation, however, is not universally accepted. At least two main rival views exist. One view is that the TPJ and STS are not specialists in social cognition; instead they play a general role related to attention.[29-32] A second alternative view is that understanding other people's minds is mediated at least partly by an entirely different mechanism called the mirror neuron system.[33] Both of these alternative views are discussed in later chapters. Given the existing evidence, however, it seems likely that the TPJ, STS, and other areas that become active during social thinking participate in some central manner in social perception and social cognition. It is to those areas that we should look first, in trying to find the attention schema.

Which Areas Might Contribute
to an Attention Schema?

Of course, I don't know where an attention schema might be implemented in the brain. If the attention schema theory is correct, if awareness is an attention schema, then that schema might be constructed mainly in one brain area, or it might be constructed by a more complex interaction among many brain areas. Maybe some or all of the STS, TPJ, and MPFC are involved. Maybe a highly localized spot in one part of the TPJ is the critical site. Maybe no one site plays a critical role, and a larger network carries out the function in aggregate. Shoehorning a function into a brain area comes with a certain intellectual risk. After all, that is how Descartes[34] made his famous mistake—chaining rational arguments, or at least arguments that seemed rational to him at the time, and concluding that the soul was located in the pineal body.

My task is, happily, a little easier than Descartes's. Much more is known about the brain now, and the function I am trying to localize is much more limited than the soul. It is an informational model of attention. Neuroscientists know more or less where informational models of color are computed, for example, or where informational models of visual motion are computed, or where informational models of sound are computed. Even something as complex and diverse as the body schema, the brain's informational model of the physical body, of its shape and movement, can be roughly attributed to a specific set of brain structures. Perhaps we have some hope of finding an approximate area or set of areas in the brain for the attention schema.

Colleagues sometimes suggest to me that a likely brain area for the attention schema might be the MPFC. I do not agree with this suggestion, as I will explain here. The MPFC is consistently recruited when people engage in social perception.[21,23–25,28,35,36] It is also active when people focus on their own thoughts and emotions.[28,36–39] The MPFC is a part of the so-called default network, a set of interconnected brain regions that are active during quiet, introspective thought, such as when people are daydreaming or replaying memories.[40,41] All of these properties together suggest that the MPFC might have something to do with self-reflection.

In my reading of the literature, however, the MPFC seems an unlikely place for the construction of an attention schema. It may be active when you are aware of yourself, but it is not terribly active when you are aware of a blue sky. Awareness itself does not seem to be related to that area of the brain. Awareness is not knowledge about yourself as a person, or knowledge about your emotions, or knowledge about your thoughts; it is not remembering your past, or introspecting about your mood, or any other part of self-reflection. Awareness is equally present whether you are reflecting on yourself or looking out at the external world. It is present whether you are focused on your innermost feelings or on the grass and sky in the park on a nice day. The MPFC may be recruited when a person introspects about his or her own thoughts and feelings, and in that sense it may play a role in conscious experience, especially in self-awareness, but it plays no obvious role in other instances of awareness. The essence of the attention schema theory, the heart of it, is that awareness is a computed model of attention. The MPFC has no particular relation to attention.

If the present theory is correct, and if a specific brain system helps to compute the attention schema, then that brain system should combine at least three key properties.

First, the system should show involvement in social perception. In particular, the system should be recruited when someone reconstructs someone else's state of attention.

Second, this hypothetical brain system should relate to one's own attention. Its activity should in some way track or reflect one's own state of attention.

Third, when that brain system is damaged, the patient should show a profound disruption in awareness. Exactly how awareness should be disrupted is difficult to predict. The symptoms would depend on how the attention schema is computed. For example, if the attention schema is computed in some map-like way, as are so many other properties in the brain, then damage to one part of the system might erase awareness of a specific part of the surrounding world.

Does any area of the brain combine these three key properties?

Both the TPJ and the STS show evidence of all three properties. They are the only brain regions that I can find in the literature that fit the description, and they fit it precisely. Of course, many other brain regions yet to be studied in detail may also fit the same description.

First, they are recruited when people are engaged in social perception. They are evidently part of the machinery for understanding the minds of others. I've briefly reviewed this involvement of the TPJ and STS in social thinking in this and previous chapters.

Second, the TPJ and STS are active when people redirect their own attention.[29-31] In some manner, these areas track one's own state of attention. This property will be described in greater detail in Chapter 16.

Third, damage to the TPJ and STS can cause a profound disruption in awareness, erasing awareness of objects in parts of space around the body.[42,43] They appear to be necessary for the brain's construction of one's own awareness. This property will be described in greater detail in Chapter 15.

In my understanding of the literature, no other brain areas satisfy all three constraints. By hypothesis, therefore, the attention schema might be dependant on these areas. The hypothesis remains uncertain. Only more experiments can fill in the details. But on the available evidence, the TPJ and STS are good candidates. They may be important nodes in a brain system that computes an attention schema.

14

The Neglect Syndrome

Can damage to a part of the brain selectively disrupt someone's awareness? Of course, awareness can be disrupted if you take a baseball bat to somebody's head. Damage to the pacemaker in your brain stem that keeps your heart and lungs going would also do the trick. But can damage to a part of the brain cause a specific, selective disruption in awareness? The clinical syndrome that comes closest is called hemispatial neglect. In this syndrome, patients suffer damage to the right side of the brain and as a result develop a difficulty in processing stimuli on the left side of space.[1,2] The reverse pattern, damage to the left side of the brain and neglect of the right side of space, is much more rare.

Neglect patients classically fail to report, react to, or notice anything in the left half of space, whether visual, auditory, tactile, or in memory. The left half of space, everything in it, any notion of performing an action in it, and any concept that it ever existed are erased from the patient's consciousness. Patients with neglect fail to dress one side of the body, fail to eat food on one side of a plate, fail to draw one side of a face when asked to copy a drawing, fail to notice or talk to people standing on the neglected side, and fail to notice that they are doing anything wrong.

Neglect is not mere blindness. People who have partial blindness, who are unable to see in a particular part of space, still know that the part of space exists and can still imagine and keep track of objects in it. Normal healthy people, for example, can have an understanding of what is directly behind them, despite having no vision behind the head. In neglect, the blindness is inside. It is a loss of awareness.

One of the more telling demonstrations of neglect involves the memory of objects.[3] In this study, a neglect patient was asked to close his eyes and imagine standing at one end of a familiar city square. When asked to describe the buildings in the square, he scanned the image in his mind and listed all the buildings to his right, neglecting the ones to his left. He did not notice that he had described only half the square. The patient was then asked to imagine that he was standing on the opposite end of the square, facing the other direction. Once again he was asked to describe the buildings, and once again he listed all the buildings to his right. This time, because he imagined facing the opposite direction, he described the opposite set of buildings and never noticed the discrepancy. He could not conceive of a left side of space. It was gone from his awareness.

Information on the left side of space can still affect the behavior of these patients. Images on the neglected side can prompt a person to say certain things or make certain choices.[4,5] For example, if a neglect patient looks at a picture of a house with flames coming out of the left-hand windows, the patient may not consciously notice the flames but may express a generally negative feeling about that particular house.[6] Somehow he or she wouldn't want to buy it or live in it. A neglect patient might flinch from a looming object on the left but deny any conscious experience of the object. When brain activity is measured in neglect patients, it turns out that the visual system still responds to the left side of space even at the highest levels of cortical processing.[7,8] The brain is clearly still processing the world on the left side. The brain is not blind to all that left-side stuff. The brain can even guide actions on the basis of objects on the left side. Yet awareness is missing.

Brain Areas Associated with Clinical Neglect

Neglect patients often have large, messy areas of damage in the brain, usually due to stroke. But by comparing across patients it is possible to find the brain area of greatest overlap, the area that, when damaged, most often results in an impairment of awareness.

Some of the brain areas associated with clinical neglect are shown in Figure 13.2. For more than half a century, neglect was thought to involve a specific area of the cerebral cortex, the posterior parietal lobe.[1,2,9] Neglect makes sense in the parietal lobe. The reason is that attention has special treatment there. Attention, as I have described in previous chapters, is a self-dynamic, a way in which some signals in the brain rise up and outcompete other signals. A network of brain areas seems to play a special role in nudging the competition, in biasing it in favor of one or another region of space. Attention, especially attention to nearby objects in specific regions of space, seems to be guided partly by a system of areas in the parietal lobe and frontal lobe that is often called the parieto-frontal attention network.[10] Neglect is classically associated with the parietal lobe, but it can also occur after lesions of the frontal lobe, though the symptoms tend to be less severe.[11–13]

These and many other findings have led to a standard interpretation of neglect. Damage to the parieto-frontal network on the right side of the brain, especially damage to the parietal lobe, causes a loss of attentional focus on the opposite side of space. Since attention can no longer be directed to anything on the left side of space, the patient fails to notice or react to objects on that side.

This standard interpretation, however, is not in perfect alignment with the data. When people with the most severe symptoms of neglect were examined, the damaged brain area was centered on the temporo-parietal junction (TPJ) in the right hemisphere.[14] Although the TPJ partially overlaps with the parietal lobe (it is after all the temporo-parietal junction), it is shifted downward in the brain from the area traditionally associated with neglect. These regions, in one example brain, are shown in Figure 13.2.

In at least one subset of neglect patients, who were considered to be especially pure in their symptoms, the most commonly damaged site was shifted even further down and forward of the TPJ, into the superior temporal sulcus (STS).[15-17] According to these studies on the TPJ and the STS, clinical neglect, especially the most severe clinical neglect, might have nothing to do with the parieto-frontal attention network. Instead, it might be associated with a swath of the cortex generally thought to be involved in social thinking.

How can the contradictions in the data be explained? To put it simply: what is neglect doing down in the STS and TPJ, when everybody knows it is supposed to be up in the parietal lobe? Where is neglect "really" centered in the brain?

The attention schema theory predicts that there should be at least two different kinds of neglect. One kind, as a primary disability, should involve difficulty *controlling* attention. This kind of neglect might be caused by damage to the parieto-frontal attention network, thought to play a role in directing the spatial locus of attention.

The second kind, as a primary disability, should involve difficulty constructing a *representation* of attention—in constructing an attention schema. This kind of neglect might be caused by damage to the TPJ or STS, thought to play a role in representing mental states.

The two predicted disabilities are not independent. Damage to one system should at least partly disrupt the other. If you damage the machinery for controlling attention, you may secondarily impair your ability to attribute awareness to yourself, since, in the present theory, awareness is a representation of attention. If you damage the machinery that attributes awareness to yourself, you may secondarily impair the control of attention, since, in the present theory, awareness synergizes with and enhances attention.

Neuroscientists now generally accept that there is no single neglect syndrome. Damage to a range of brain areas can cause neglect, and different neglect patients can have somewhat different mixtures of symptoms.[15,17-20] It is therefore not correct to attribute all forms of neglect to a single brain area or mechanism. The present theory suggests a complex, interconnected system with many components and at least two different flavors of neglect. Yet despite the complexity of the literature, one central coincidence stands out: clinical neglect is most severe after damage to the right TPJ, and the right TPJ participates in social thinking—in constructing models of minds. This coincidence, so puzzling from a traditional point of view, makes sense in the context of the attention schema theory.

Challenge 1: Loss of Awareness Is Not the Only Symptom of Clinical Neglect

As I noted throughout previous chapters, I received a great deal of feedback from colleagues on the attention schema theory. Much of that feedback was enthusiastic, some of it challenging, and all of it helpful in forcing me to think deeply about all aspects of the theory. In the remainder of this chapter I will describe three particular challenges to the theory. These challenges concern the relationship between the attention schema theory and the clinical syndrome of neglect. In each case I will describe the challenge as it was presented to me, and then I will provide a possible answer.

One challenge to my proposal could be put this way.[21] I am proposing that clinical neglect is, at root, a loss of awareness. You lose awareness of objects on the left side of space. But why would a loss of awareness cause you to stop reacting to those objects? Wouldn't you keep on reacting to those objects normally, but simply have no awareness that you were doing it? In neglect, you don't merely lose awareness of objects on the left; you generally also stop reacting to them.

Patients do sometimes react to objects on the neglected side. For example, a patient might duck from an incoming ball without any awareness that there was a ball or that there was a left side of space for the ball to be moving through. But most of the time, neglect patients react to objects on the right and fail to react to anything on the left. Therefore, according to this challenge, clinical neglect cannot be explained as a left-sided gap in awareness. It is a disability in the control of behavior.

This counterargument is based on a common notion about awareness. In that notion, awareness is an epiphenomenon. As an epiphenomenon, awareness should be a feeling that serves no function and has no effect on behavior. It should merely come along for the ride, having no impact on the machine. In the epiphenomenon view, a person without awareness would indeed act normally and lack only the inner experience. Take away awareness of objects on the left side of space, and the person should still act in an outwardly normal way.

The epiphenomenon view, however, is logically impossible. We can say we are aware; therefore, awareness can affect at least one kind of behavior, namely speech. Since awareness is not an epiphenomenon, since it plays a role in controlling at least some behavior, damaging awareness should have a measurable impact on behavior. In the present theory, awareness is an informational model constructed in the brain. That model has a use. It is constructed for the purpose of guiding behavior. Losing awareness of objects in the left half of space should alter a person's behavior toward those objects.

In the attention schema theory, a natural resonance exists between awareness and attention. Awareness and attention are situated something like two mirrors facing each other. Each enhances the other. Because of this resonance, awareness must profoundly influence attention. Without awareness of an object, attention to that object should be deflated. Without attention, behavioral reactions should be vastly reduced. In this theory, therefore, the symptoms of neglect as they are typically described—no awareness of objects on the left, reduced ability to direct attention toward the left, *and* little tendency to react to objects on the left—are the expected result of damaging the attention schema.

Challenge 2: Why Don't People with Neglect Also Have a Disability in Social Perception?

A second common challenge to my proposal goes as follows. Suppose I am right. Suppose that awareness is constructed by the social machinery. Suppose that damage to the social machinery disrupts awareness and causes clinical neglect. Then why aren't patients with neglect also socially impaired? People with neglect can carry on a conversation anyway, even if they typically show some confusion. In what sense is neglect explainable as a failure of the social machinery? No failure of the social machinery is evident (according to this argument, anyway).

The simplest answer to this challenge is that patients with clinical neglect probably *do* have social disabilities. Damage to the right TPJ and STS causes a disability in social thinking, at least as reported in some case studies.[22–24]

To test the relationship systematically, one would have to look to the correct patient subpopulation. Neglect caused by parieto-frontal damage may spare the social machinery. People with that flavor of neglect may have no social deficits. In contrast, neglect caused by damage to the STS or TPJ ought to disrupt social cognition. Failure to select the correct patient population would obscure the result.

One would also have to test the correct subset of social abilities. If my proposal is correct, then neglect is caused by damaging a part of the attention schema. As a result, a neglect patient cannot construct his or her own awareness of the left side of space. The corresponding social deficit associated with neglect should be a difficulty in attributing someone else's awareness to that same side of space. No other social capability need be damaged, although, depending on how large and messy the brain lesion is, other symptoms might join in.

Challenge 3: Why Does Neglect Affect Only One Side of Space?

A third common challenge to the attention schema theory is much harder to answer. Why is neglect one-sided? Why do people lose awareness on the left and not on the right? If the attention schema theory explains some aspects of neglect, then how does it explain that particular aspect?

I do not think anyone fully understands why neglect typically affects the left side of space and rarely affects the right. Hypotheses abound and certainties are absent. It is my opinion that the true reason has yet to be discovered.

If consciousness were a Cartesian thing, a unified spirit not of this world, then we might be concerned about its apparent division in neglect. Descartes, after all, was certain that consciousness was a unified thing that couldn't be housed in two separate containers in the brain. However, if awareness is a computed property, an informational model, then there is no reason to suppose that the model stands or falls in one piece. Evidently it is possible to muck up the computations regarding one half of space while sparing the other half of space. If the attention schema theory is correct, if machinery somewhere in the brain computes a model of attention, then that machinery apparently has some map-like physical layout to it. It is possible to damage one part of that map while leaving the rest functionally intact.

Consider a more traditional view of consciousness. Suppose that awareness is a direct emanation, or aura, or consequence of the processing of information in the brain. In that case, it is difficult to understand why a hole in the middle of the right hemisphere should erase awareness of *everything* in the left half of space. Most of the right hemisphere is still capable of processing information. The visual system, for example, is still active—the neurons are still actively processing images from the left side of space.[7] Why is that information no longer generating consciousness? What happened to the awareness generated by the visual information in visual cortex, or the awareness generated by tactile information in somatosensory cortex? Why has that awareness gone away? Given that patients can still process information from the left, process it deeply, and have that information affect their behavior, where did the awareness of that information go?

In contrast, if the present approach is correct and awareness is a computed representation, then losing awareness of half of space can be explained naturally. The syndrome is something like losing color perception in a part of space. If you damage your color-computing machinery for a part of the visual world, you can still compute other information, but you can't attach the property of color to it. You become colorblind for part of space. Likewise, if you damage the specific machinery that computes the feature of awareness, then you can still compute other information but can't attach awareness to it. You become awareness-blind for part of space.

The attention schema theory, therefore, gives quite a reasonable explanation for why neglect might affect one side of space and not the other. But why does neglect affect the *left* side of space in particular, and so rarely the right? The answer is that nobody knows. The left-sided nature of neglect is one of its most consistent features and one of the most puzzling. Damage certain areas of the right hemisphere and awareness of the left half of space is erased. You would think the mirror image would result, that damaging the same areas in the left hemisphere would erase awareness of the right half of space. But this is almost never so.

In the most common speculation,[12,25,26] the machinery that allows for awareness is so much weaker or smaller in the left hemisphere that damaging it has little noticeable effect. The other side can take over. The corresponding machinery in the right hemisphere is so dominant that when it is damaged, the system tries to compensate but can't entirely—hence clinical neglect. Other explanations have also been suggested involving a competition between the two hemispheres.[27,28]

Exactly why neglect is usually left-sided remains to be settled but appears to be a matter of specific implementation—of exactly how the hardware is distributed in the brain. The important point with respect to the attention schema theory is that the essential properties of neglect, the loss of awareness for a part of space, the damage to an area of the brain that otherwise seems to participate in social perception—these properties make a certain sense in the context of the theory.

15

Multiple Interlocking Functions of the Brain Area TPJ

In the previous chapter I pointed out a strange coincidence, if it is a coincidence. A region of the brain, encompassing the temporo-parietal junction (TPJ) and superior temporal sulcus (STS), is active during social thinking. This brain region is recruited when people think about other people's minds. Yet the same general region of the brain, when damaged, can cause a devastating disruption in one's own awareness of the world. It can cause clinical neglect. To me, the overlap of these two properties provided an initial clue. It suggested a deep connection between social thinking and awareness. It suggested that just as we use our social intelligence to attribute awareness to someone else, we may also attribute awareness to ourselves. Awareness itself may be a construct computed by some part of the social machinery.

For the past twenty years, however, the possible relationship between social perception and clinical neglect has been ignored. These functions are generally treated as though they belong to unrelated scientific disciplines. They have been placed in separate boxes and have separate experimental literatures. The inconvenient overlap is often dismissed. The TPJ can't be related to clinical neglect because everybody knows it's really a social area. The TPJ can't be a social area because everybody knows it's related to clinical neglect. Every possible intellectual crowbar has been used to pry apart the social functions and clinical neglect. I think it may be time to stop trying to separate those functions and consider the possibility that they are somehow related.

Over the years, more findings have accumulated about the STS and TPJ, and each new discovery has tended to spark a round of confusion and skepticism. The TPJ in particular is piling up function after function. Either it is a cortical Rorschach, revealing any function you choose to see in it, or its many disparate functions are related in some deep manner that is not generally appreciated. To me, these many functions point clearly in one direction. They point toward the attention schema theory. They point toward awareness as a specific aspect of computing models of minds.

In the following sections I briefly note three additional properties of the TPJ and STS that point in that direction.

The Ventral Attention System

Attention is a competition among signals in the brain. The competition fluctuates as various signals rise up in strength and then sink down again to give play to other signals. Attention has a self-dynamic. It can, however, be guided by specific control signals in the brain. These control signals do not entirely dictate the state of attention. Instead, they bias it. They help to shape the ongoing competition. In a now well-accepted view that I discussed in previous chapters, these biasing signals that help to guide attention are generated mainly in the parietal and frontal lobes, in the so-called parieto-frontal attention network.

One set of experiments, however, obtained surprising results that seemed to conflict with the traditional view. When a person's attention was shifted to a new location, especially to a sudden or unexpected stimulus, the brain showed elevated activity in a set of areas including the TPJ, some parts of the STS, and a region in the lower part of the frontal lobe.[1-3] The brain activity was strongest in the right hemisphere.

Is the TPJ related to social thinking or to attention? In the attention schema theory, the attentional functions and the social functions are not in contradiction. One of the fundamental points of this theory is that modeling attention is an important part of modeling a mind. To understand and predict the behavior of another person, it is useful to model that person's attentional dynamics. To understand and predict one's own behavior, it is useful to model one's own attentional dynamics. In this theory, the regions of the brain involved in social perception should also be involved in tracking or monitoring or modeling one's own attention.

It has been argued that the two functions, the attention functions and the social cognition functions, are represented in separate areas in the TPJ that happen to be so near each other that the brain scanning techniques have blurred them. For example, one functional imaging study found that attention tasks and social cognition tasks recruited overlapping areas of activity in the TPJ, but the areas of activation had distinct, spatially separated peaks.[4]

This attempt to separate the "attention" subarea of the TPJ from the "social" subarea, however, does not entirely address the underlying issue. The cortex is generally organized by functional proximity. Similar or related functions tend to be processed near each other,[5,6] presumably so that they can better connect and interact with each other. This trend toward functional clustering seems to hold true in the social domain. Rather than view the proximity of different functions such as attention and social cognition as a contradiction, or suggest that one function must be correct and the other a mistake, or suggest that the functions must be separate from each other and co-localized merely as an accident of brain organization, I am suggesting here that the functions interact and are therefore not mutually contradictory.

Autobiographical Memory and the TPJ

When people reminisce, recalling specific memories from their own past lives, a widespread set of brain areas is typically active, among them, consistently, the TPJ.[7-9]

This apparent involvement of the TPJ with autobiographical memory provides another piece of the larger puzzle. In the attention schema theory, awareness is a constructed feature, a bundle of information, that can be bound to other information in the brain. One type of information particularly relevant to consciousness is self-knowledge—not just knowledge of your physical body, not just knowledge of your current emotions and thoughts, but also your autobiographical memories that help to define your sense of personhood and your sense of continuity through time. In the present theory, autobiographical memories are not a part of awareness itself. But they can be linked to awareness. They help define the "I" in "I am aware of X." Whatever computes the proposed attention schema, it should have a special relationship to autobiographical memory.

The Out-of-Body Experience

The very existence of an out-of-body illusion could be interpreted as evidence in support of the attention schema theory, for the following reasons. Assume for a moment that this theory is wrong and that awareness is not computed information. Suppose instead that awareness is an emergent property, a byproduct of neuronal activity. Neurons compute information and as a result, somehow, awareness of that information occurs. In that case, why would we feel the awareness as located in, and emanating from, our own selves? By what mechanism does the awareness feel as though it is anchored here or anywhere else? In the out-of-body illusion, why do we feel as though awareness has been shifted to a new, specific location? Why is awareness given any location at all? If awareness emerges from information, and the information is computed by a machine, and the machine happens to be in a certain location, by what logic does the awareness feel like it comes from that location? The fact that awareness "feels" like it is in a specific location suggests that it is a computed model that includes a computed spatial structure.

What regions in the brain might compute this spatial aspect of awareness? The out-of-body illusion can be evoked by electrically disrupting the TPJ in the right hemisphere.[10] Evidently, the right TPJ is crucial for computing the spatial structure of awareness.

Overview of the Many Interlocking Functions

A suspiciously large set of functions has been attributed to the TPJ and STS in the right hemisphere, especially to the TPJ. Consider the list:

   The TPJ is involved in social cognition, especially in reconstructing the beliefs of other people.[11-16] The STS is also involved in some aspects of social perception. It is recruited when the brain processes the intentional actions of others, such as reaching, grasping, or looking.[17-23]

   The TPJ and STS become active when you switch attention to a new item.[1-3] Activity in these brain areas not only reflects your understanding of other people's minds but also reflects your own state of attention.

   Damage to the TPJ and STS on the right side of the brain can sometimes lead to a profound neglect of everything on the left side of space.[24,25] This neglect, caused by TPJ and STS damage, is the most devastating derangement of awareness known in the clinical literature.

   The TPJ is involved in computing the spatial locus of one's own mind. Scrambling its signals through electrical stimulation can result in an out-of-body experience.[10]

   The TPJ is consistently recruited when people recall autobiographical memories.[7-9]

Given these many findings, the general region of the TPJ and STS on the right side of the brain seems suspiciously like a magic area that does everything. The good, skeptical scientist is tempted to conclude that the experimental work must be misguided or misinterpreted. Too much is being attributed to one spot in the brain. These many functions have occasioned a certain amount of controversy. Consider a partial list of controversies:

Traditionally, attention to the space around the body is controlled by the parieto-frontal network. But why do attention-related tasks also activate the TPJ and STS? Where exactly is spatial attention controlled?

Traditionally, clinical neglect is caused by damage to the parietal lobe. But the most severe cases of neglect are centered on the TPJ. The TPJ overlaps with the parietal lobe but it is mainly outside the region traditionally associated with clinical neglect. How can the discrepancy in localization be reconciled? This discrepancy is so inconvenient that it is often simply ignored.

What does the out-of-body experience have to do with any of these other functions?

What do any of these functions have to do with recalling personal memories?

Where in all the scattered mess of scientific findings does awareness fit in, and what is the practical difference between awareness and attention?

The attention schema theory extracts some order out of the chaos. The brain uses the process of attention in order to sort data—to focus on some signals at the expense of other signals. In the theory, the brain also computes an attention schema. That schema is a descriptive model of attention. It is used in social perception to monitor and predict someone else's state of attention, in effect attributing awareness to another person. It is also used to model one's own attention, in effect attributing awareness to oneself. The TPJ may be a critical brain node for computing this attention schema. Many of the properties ascribed to the TPJ—constructing models of other people's beliefs, tracking one's own attention, triggering clinical neglect when damaged, participating in the out-of-body experience, becoming active in association with autobiographical memory—are consistent with constructing an attention schema and attributing awareness to others and to oneself. The pieces, drawn from a great variety of subdisciplines and brain systems, from lesion studies, behavioral studies, brain imaging studies, and even monkey physiology studies, fit together. In my own laboratory at Princeton we continue to study the human TPJ and other brain regions to understand how an attention schema might be instantiated in the brain and how it might be responsible for awareness.

16

Simulating Other Minds

Humans are social animals. We are experts at navigating a complex social world. But how is social intelligence built into the brain?

Neuroscientists have proposed two main views. The first view, summarized in the previous chapters, is that social capability depends on an expert brain system. That brain system includes the temporo-parietal junction (TPJ), the superior temporal sulcus (STS), and many other interconnected regions. This brain system can compute useful, predictive models of other people's minds. The main evidence to support this view is that the same, consistent set of brain areas becomes active when people engage in a great variety of social thinking.

The second view of how social capability is built into the brain is called simulation theory. In simulation theory, social perception is essentially the result of empathy. We have an innate, direct understanding of ourselves, of our own motives, emotions, and experiences. We understand other people's minds by reference to our own internal experiences. In effect, we put ourselves in other people's shoes.

These two views of social perception, the expert system view and the simulation view, are often considered to be rival explanations.

In the previous chapters I discussed the expert system view and how it may relate to the attention schema theory. If the brain does compute something like an attention schema, it may do so through its expert system in social perception, and brain areas TPJ and STS seem to be crucial nodes in that computation. But how does the attention schema theory relate to the simulation view of social perception? Since it is compatible with the expert system view, is it therefore necessarily incompatible with the simulation view?

In this chapter I argue that, actually, the attention schema theory is compatible with both of the rival views—the expert system view and the simulation view of social perception. Moreover, I suggest that these two rival views of social perception shouldn't be rivals, that they are compatible with each other, and that the brain probably uses both methods in a hybrid system to make us socially capable beings. That hybrid system may solve some of the difficulties of each approach by itself.

Mirror Neurons

The experimental heart of simulation theory is the phenomenon of mirror neurons. Rizzolatti and colleagues first discovered mirror neurons in the premotor cortex of macaque monkeys.[1-3]

The experimenters were studying a region of cortex involved in controlling the hand during grasping. Neurons in this brain area became active during particular, complex types of grasp. For example, one neuron might become active when the monkey reached out to pick up a raisin using a precision grip between the thumb and forefinger. Another neuron might become active during a power grip that required the whole hand. In the course of studying these motor neurons, the experimenters made an unexpected discovery. Sometimes the experimenter grasped an object in front of the monkey in order to move it into or out of reach. Strangely, some of the monkey's own motor neurons became active at the sight of the experimenter's grasp. The mirror neurons, as they came to be called, had both motor and sensory properties. They responded regardless of whether the monkey performed or saw a particular action.

Mirror-like properties were then reported in the human cortex. Volunteers were placed in an MRI scanner and either performed a hand action or watched a hand action. A specific set of areas in the cortex became active in both conditions.[4–6] Humans and monkeys seemed to have a similar mirror-neuron network, spanning areas of the parietal lobe, the premotor cortex, and the STS.[7]

The hypothesized role of mirror neurons is to aid in understanding the actions of others. In that hypothesis, we understand someone else's hand actions by activating our own hand-control machinery and in that way covertly simulating the actions. The mirror-neuron hypothesis is in some ways an elaboration of Liberman's older and, alas, rarely credited hypothesis about speech comprehension.[8] In that hypothesis, we understand someone else's speech sounds by using our own motor machinery to mimic the same sounds in a subtle, subvocal manner.

Mirror neurons have been studied almost exclusively in the context of hand actions—performing them and perceiving them. Consequently, the "mirror-neuron network" is suspiciously similar to the network of brain areas involved in planning hand actions. This limitation is probably a mistake, and the idea of mirror neurons residing in a limited network is also probably a mistake. The concept of mirroring can in principle be generalized beyond the perception of other people's hand actions to all social perception and to a great variety of brain areas.

When you see someone getting hit in the face with a baseball, you tend to cringe sympathetically. Are your mirror neurons generating the same facial action you would make if you were hit? When you watch a boxing match you tend to make subtle punching movements. When you see someone else smile you are more likely to smile. Even beyond simple actions, you may understand the pain of someone else's stubbed toe by using your own somatosensory system to imagine the pain. You may understand someone else's joy, complete with nuances and psychological implications, by using your own emotional machinery to simulate that joy. You may understand someone else's intellectual point of view by activating a version of that point of view in your own brain. You may understand other minds in general by simulating them using the same machinery within your own brain. The entire brain may be a simulator of other brains. In this way we could, according to simulation theory, gain insight into others by putting ourselves in other people's shoes.

Difficulties with the Mirror-Neuron Story

The mirror-neuron story is still controversial. The experimental support is far from complete. Perhaps the greatest weakness in the mirror-neuron story right now is that the experimental support is still circumstantial. The results are mainly correlative. Mirror neurons may be active when you watch someone else's behavior; but do mirror neurons actually *cause* you to understand someone else's behavior?

Alternative views of mirror neurons have been offered. For example, perhaps the purpose of mirror neurons is not to understand the actions of others but to facilitate imitation. We learn by imitation; perhaps we are wired to translate sight into action. After all, monkeys are good at imitation but rather poor at social cognition compared to humans, and monkeys have plenty of mirror neurons.

Another alternative interpretation of mirror neurons, recently suggested, is that they are a byproduct without any specific function, merely a symptom of the frequent association between the sight of the hand and the control of the hand.[9,10] Every time you grasp something you also see yourself do it, and by association, by repetition, neurons in areas scattered throughout the brain may become entrained to respond to both conditions. In this view, mirror neurons are not part of any machinery for social perception. Instead, they are a meaningless symptom of other more important functions.

This debate about mirror neurons can only be resolved by further experiments and especially by more direct experiments. To support the mirror-neuron story, an experiment will need to be done in which the mirror neurons are temporarily disrupted. As a result, the person or monkey should have a specific, temporary drop in ability to understand the actions of others. Another experimental approach might be to electrically excite a small clump of mirror neurons in person A, say a clump of mirror neurons that encodes a precision grip, and then determine if person A is more likely to think that person B has made a precision grip. The mirror-neuron story needs a direct link showing that mirror neurons *cause* social perception. With that direct link established, it would then be possible to move forward and work out exactly how mirror neurons contribute to social perception. To be fair, however, the complaint that "it needs more data" could be leveled against almost any theory out there.

The mirror-neuron story has had an immense impact on neuroscience, psychology, and philosophy. Simulation theory provides deep insight into how people go about understanding people, how people empathize with each other, and how under some circumstances people may *fail* to empathize with each other. The theoretical implications are huge. Yet simulation theory suffers from two main gaps in its logic that are commonly noted. I will briefly describe them in the following sections. To be clear, I am not arguing against the mirror-neuron story. I find it extremely interesting and of great potential importance. It deservedly remains an area of active research. In the following sections I focus on certain logical gaps in the theory because I believe the gaps can be closed. The difficulties can be resolved by combining simulation theory with the expert system approach to social cognition. The two methods, working together, get around the obstacles.

Difficulty 1: No Clear Labeling of Individuals

In simulation theory, you understand someone else's thoughts, emotions, and actions by activating the same machinery in your own brain. But the theory does not provide any obvious way to distinguish your own thoughts, intentions, and emotions from someone else's. Both are run on the same hardware. If the simulation theory is strictly true, then how can I tell the difference between my own inner experiences and someone else's that I am simulating? For that matter, if I am in a room with five other people, if I am engaged in social perception and social cognition, building an understanding of their minds and motives, then how can I tell which mental states belong to which people? If motivations and thoughts, intentions and actions are all simulated on the same hardware in my brain, then how can I sort what belongs to whom?

Difficulty 2: Circularity

Simulation theory, at least in its simplest form, is circular. The essential idea is that to know someone else's state of mind, you re-create that state of mind in yourself. But how can you re-create a state of mind if you don't already know what it is? Before Brain A can mirror the state of Brain B, it needs to know what state to mirror. Brain A needs a mechanism that generates hypotheses about the state of Brain B.

A Hybrid System: Combining Mirror Neurons with the Expert System

The two conceptual difficulties with simulation theory disappear in a hybrid system that combines both approaches, the simulation approach and the expert system approach to social perception.

In the hybrid system proposed here, the brain contains an expert system. This system probably includes the standard brain areas that light up in most experiments on social cognition, such as the TPJ, STS, and medial prefrontal cortex (MPFC). This system uses a convergence of information—how other people look and act, how they sound, prior information about them, their words, their gestures.

The expert system, combining this information, constructs models of other minds. These models include reconstructions of the beliefs of others, the thoughts of others, the emotions of others, the intentions to make this or that movement, the goals of behavior, the state of another person's attention, and so on.

These models of minds are in essence elaborate hypotheses. They can be used to drive mirror-neuron networks that span much of the brain and that simulate and thereby refine the hypotheses. In this speculation, models of minds are constructed or coordinated by a restricted network of areas specialized in social intelligence, the network that is so commonly recruited when people engage in social thinking. That network is in a constant dialogue with a mirror-neuron system that includes most of the rest of the brain.

The hybrid model makes a specific set of predictions. If your premotor hand area is damaged, you should still be able to perceive the hand actions of others. But the details and nuances, the mechanics of hand action, should be harder to understand. If your visual machinery is damaged, you should still be able to understand the concept of someone else seeing something. But the details and nuances should escape you. If you have deficient emotional circuitry, you should be able to understand that someone else is experiencing emotion, but the richness and nuance of that social understanding should be compromised. Losing the simulation machinery should not remove basic social perception or cognition, the ability to generate basic hypotheses about what other people are experiencing, but should limit the detail and richness of the perceptual models.

One of the nagging difficulties of the expert system view of social thinking is that the expert system would need to be an expert on rather a large range of topics. Is the other person aware of that coffee cup? The social machinery must be informed about coffee cups. Is she aware of the chill in the room? The social machinery must be informed about skin temperature. Is she aware of the abstract idea that I am trying to get across, or is she distracted by her own thoughts? What emotion is she feeling? What movement is she planning? Why does her voice sound too loud? Why did she move so quickly? Why did she choose one cut of clothes over another? Social perception requires an extraordinary multimodal linkage of information. All things sensory, emotional, cognitive, intellectual, cultural, or action oriented must be brought together and considered in order to build a useful predictive model of the other person's mind. It is implausible to talk about a specific expert region of the brain that performs all of social perception.

In the hybrid system proposed here, the expert system does not need to be omniscient. It does not need to duplicate, in miniature, the expertise of the entire brain. The mirror-neuron phenomenon provides the diversity and computing power. During social perception, to understand what another person is seeing, the brain recruits visual areas; to understand what another person is doing, the brain recruits motor areas; to understand what another person is feeling, the brain recruits emotional processors; but at the center of this vast brain-wide network lies a restricted set of areas, specialists in social cognition. These areas coordinate the perceptual model of a mind, generate the initial hypotheses, and drive the mirror-neuron simulations.

Difficulty 1: Solving the Labeling of Individuals

When we human think about each other, we do not conceive of a mind as merely a collection of emotions, motivations, and thoughts. We conceive of a mind as a thing that resides here or there, in a particular location. A perceptual model of a mind includes, among its many components, a spatial location assigned to the model. It is true perception in the sense that the perceived properties have a perceived location to form a perceived object. This spatial embodiment is especially apparent in the out-of-body experience. In that state, the machinery has been disrupted and the brain computes and assigns an incorrect location to one's own mind. My thoughts, my emotions, my motivations, my intentions—these are all suddenly located in the upper corner of the room. Or seem to be.

This spatial embodiment of a mind is evidently a function of an expert system. In the now classic experiment by Blanke and colleagues,[11] disruption of the TPJ in the right hemisphere caused an out-of-body experience. Vesting a mind with a location, with a spatial structure, may be a part of the building of models carried out by the TPJ and perhaps other areas in the social cognition network.

We don't normally think of social perception as being literally like sensory perception. But in this sense it is: we construct a set of properties and bind them to a spatial location. This ability to compute a spatial embodiment when constructing a model of a mind solves one of the long-standing difficulties of simulation theory. You know whether the perceived mental states are yours, or John's, or Susan's, in the same way that you know whether the color blue belongs to your shirt, to John's shirt, to Susan's shirt, or to the car at the curb. You keep track of it by spatial assignment. You perceive the thoughts and emotions to be emanating spatially from this person, that person, or from yourself. A model of a mind comes with a spatial assignment. Simulation theory by itself cannot solve the problem, but combined with a computed model of a mind, complete with a computed spatial structure, that particular problem disappears.

Difficulty 2: Solving Circularity

Before Brain A can mirror the state of Brain B, it needs to know what state to mirror. Brain A needs a mechanism that generates hypotheses about the state of Brain B. What generates the initial hypotheses?

In the hybrid model proposed here, specialized areas generate the hypotheses about other people's mind states. Those hypotheses are further refined by simulation. If you look at another person grasping a pen, first visual information enters the eye, percolates through the visual system, and reaches the biological motion neurons in the STS. This expert system in the STS uses incoming visual information to categorize the action. The biological motion detectors in the STS are, essentially, computing a hypothesis about the nature of the action. The STS can then drive the mirror neurons that simulate the action. The mirror neurons essentially compute the details of how you would perform the action. The simulation provides nuanced information about the action. In this way, your understanding of the other person's action is built up by a dialogue between an expert system and a mirror-neuron system. The likely dependence of mirror neurons on an interaction with the STS has been emphasized before.[7]

In the hybrid system, mirror neurons are not rivals to the theory that social perception is emphasized in specialized regions such as the TPJ and STS. Instead, the two mechanisms for social perception could operate in a cooperative fashion. In this proposed scheme, the mirror-neuron system is an extended loop adding to and enhancing the machinery that constructs models of minds.

Simulation of One's Own Mind: The Resonance Loop

In the previous section I discussed the possibility that social perception includes two interrelated processes: constructing a model of a mind, and elaborating on that model through brain-wide simulation. The separation between these two processes is probably artificial or at least less categorical than the labels suggest. Think how much more complicated, in a recursive, loop-the-loop way, these processes become when applied to oneself.

Suppose that you are modeling your own mind state. Suppose your self model includes the hypothesis that you are angry right now. To enhance that hypothesis, to enrich the details through simulation, the machinery that constructs your self model contacts and uses your emotion-generating machinery. The state of anger is implemented there. In that case, if you weren't actually angry, the mirroring process should make you become so as a side product. If you were already angry, perhaps you become more so.

Suppose your self model includes the self prediction that you might reach out and pick up a cup of juice. To enrich that model through simulation, the machinery that constructs the model contacts and uses your motor machinery to simulate the action, thereby priming the action and making you more likely to actually do it.

In each case, what the self model depicts becomes more likely to pass. The self model is not merely an after-the-fact reconstruction but also has the power to control the system. The reason is that the self model uses the system as an extension of itself. The self model and the self that is being modeled are intertwined.

In this hypothesis, a fundamental difference exists between constructing a model of someone else's mind and constructing a model of your own mind. In constructing a model of someone else's mind, there is no direct mechanism for that model to alter the other person's mind. The loop is open, not closed. There is no resonance. But in constructing a model of your own mind, the model alters the thing that it depicts. The model is both a perceptual representation and an executive controller. It is a description and an actor. It is like the mission statement of a company that, by describing the company, makes it so.

I have not gone beyond the attention schema theory of consciousness proposed in the earlier chapters of the book. Awareness is proposed to be an informational model of attention. The theory remains mechanistic. In principle, it could be built into an electronic circuit. It contains no magic. And yet by considering more and more of the implementation details, and more and more of the recursive complexities that might result from that implementation, the theoretical description of a conscious mind begins to sound more like the intuitive notion that we all have based on introspection. Consciousness is both an observer of the world in us and around us, and also a controller.

17

Some Spiritual Matters

If a scientist discovers a bird or a monkey in the wild behaving irrationally and doing so persistently, the light of enthusiasm will enter that scientist's eye. How can we understand the creature's irrational behavior? Can we study it from an evolutionary, a biological, a neuroscientific point of view? What environmental forces led to that behavior pattern? Does the behavior, after all, have a hidden use? Even if it is costly to the animal, would rewiring or relearning be even more costly?

When a scientist observes humans behaving irrationally, especially if the irrationality has anything to do with religion, suddenly the science goes out the window. The desire to understand a natural phenomenon is gone. The reaction is one of derision and contempt. It reeks of moral superiority, as though the scientist, failing utterly in even the most basic modicum of self-awareness, were proclaiming, "Myself, I have no irrationalities to speak of. The rest of the world should, for its own sake, be as rational as I am."

I was brought up in the scientific and atheistic fold and still consider myself a scientist first and an atheist second. The one leads to the other. Perhaps I can be forgiven for providing some gentle criticism to my own kind. Science is about gaining insight into the world. Neuroscience is about gaining insight into the brain and how it guides behavior. And spirituality and religion are nonignorable large components of human behavior. How can we, as scientists, turn our backs on these phenomena? If they are irrational, they are also ubiquitous and must have some scientific or naturalistic explanation. We will never truly understand this side of human behavior if, in studying it, we set ourselves the agenda of belittling it.

The past ten years have seen a rapid growth in the cognitive science of religion, the study of religion as a natural phenomenon that can be understood from the point of view of psychology, neuroscience, and especially evolution. Among those who have contributed to this field are Dennett,[1] Boyer,[2] Barrett,[3] Atran,[4] Sosis and colleagues,[5] and many others. This area of study finally takes religion seriously as a biological phenomenon worth studying at a mechanistic level.

Lately, when I give scientific talks at academic departments, I find that I run myself into trouble. The reason is that, by talking about consciousness, I am often led through question-and-answer to the topic of spirituality. Spirituality is, literally, about spirits. We humans see spirit in ourselves, in other people, in our pets, and sometimes, depending on who you are talking to, in the inanimate objects around us, or in the spaces around us, or in the universe as a whole. The spirit world is the world of perceived consciousness. How many times have you gotten mad at your car because it won't start? How many children perceive a soul in a stuffed animal? How many people believe in a deistic mind, an omnipotent awareness? Consciousness, especially our human tendency to attribute consciousness to the things around us, provides the stuff of the spirit world. Talk about consciousness and you soon begin to talk about spiritual belief.

Yet the scientific study of spirituality and religiosity is not as widely recognized as it ought to be. To talk about spirituality or religion to a roomful of scientists, you are expected to start with a disclaimer, a clear statement of allegiance. The audience expects you to announce, either in words or tone of voice, "I don't believe in the silliness, religion is the cause of most social ills, and I am about to denigrate it." Having communicated your loyalties and reassured the audience, you are then accepted into the group and the audience is willing to listen to your scientific story.

My difficulty is that I do not have so negative a view of human spiritual or religious behavior. I am an atheist in the literal sense—I do not believe that an actual deity created the universe (or created anything at all). I do not believe in spirits that are separate from the machinery of the brain. Like many scientists I think consciousness is a construction of the human brain. Disembodied spirits therefore do not exist, and no minds of any kind existed before the evolution of the brain. However, an intensively human phenomenon exists—spirituality. It reminds me of music, another complex and intensively human phenomenon, also completely irrational, that is an important part of my own life. The amount of mental calories I've burnt on playing and composing music over the course of my life is incredible. If I can have my music then I don't begrudge people their religion. I would rather study it as a fascinating part of the natural world than preach against it.

I think it is easy for the atheistic side to point to an extreme segment of religion, that fifteen or twenty percent that are so dogmatic, so shrill, and so afraid of intellectual enlightenment that they harm the rest of us. Religion can be terribly destructive. But the vast majority of people belong to a different religious mindset. The moderate religious are too often forgotten in the culture-war debates. They compose the bulk of the human population. Most people that I've talked to are curious about the world around them. They want to know. They welcome insight into the deep questions. Who are we, where did we come from, what happens when we die, what is a mind, can it exist independently of a physical body, is there a higher intelligence that governs it all or are we the highest intelligence in the neighborhood?

When moderate people look to the more extreme religious leaders, the answers are not satisfactory. Too much certainty. Too much blind trust required. And somehow the blind trust ends up benefitting the leaders themselves, usually financially. So people turn to science. I believe most people are fascinated by what science might tell us about the deep philosophical questions. The difficulty is that science has some of the same bad habits. Too much outward certainty. Too little consideration for people's cultural choices. The attitude needlessly turns people away.

For all these reasons I would like to say here that I do not claim to have the answers to the deep questions. Scientific certainty is not possible. Moreover, by explaining consciousness in a mechanistic fashion, I am not attempting to do away with spirituality. In the theory described in this book, spirit is information in the brain and therefore literally exists. I accept the usefulness—the cultural usefulness, the humanistic usefulness, the personal usefulness—of considering spiritual questions.

Having a specific theory of consciousness, of what a spirit actually *is*, brings with it a certain advantage. I can apply the theory to many of the popular, deep, philosophical questions and see what answers arise. I cannot pretend to answer these questions definitively. I do not know the answers. But I can reason from my proposed theory of consciousness and see where it leads me.

In this chapter I apply the attention schema theory to several frequently asked, fundamental questions.

Free Will

Do humans have free will?

I confess to a certain cringe reflex when encountering that trite old question. I will say nothing about Newtonian determinism, quantum mechanical uncertainty, compatibilists and incompatibilists, or any other common approach. Instead, I am going to focus on one question: according to the attention schema theory, does consciousness have any control over our behavior?

One view of consciousness is that it is an epiphenomenon. It is a side product of the brain, just like heat is a side product of the hardware in a computer. Consciousness rides on top of the neural computations, but it has no physical capacity to impact behavior. In other words, consciousness *is* but doesn't *do*. In this view, consciousness thinks it has free will but is mistaken. Conscious control, conscious decision, conscious intention, are all illusion.

In a closely related view, consciousness is a story that we invent to make sense of our behavior after the fact. This "after-the-fact" hypothesis harks back at least to Gazzaniga's interpreter,[6] the hypothetical brain system in each of us that invents a personal narrative. Nisbett and Wilson[7] made a similar proposal in which consciousness is the brain's often wrong reconstruction of what it is doing and why. Perhaps the best known example of this type of hypothesis comes from Libet and colleagues,[8] who claimed that when people perform an action, the plan to move is generated first and the conscious intention to act is generated shortly thereafter. Libet and colleagues suggested that conscious intention does not actually cause people to perform an action; instead, it is a way to make sense of the action after the fact.

In this after-the-fact hypothesis, consciousness does have some impact on behavior. It provides a person with information on the self (albeit information that is reconstructed and sometimes inaccurate). That information can be used to shape future behavior. At the very least, that information can help us talk our way out of trouble, explaining our bad behavior afterward. However, the impact of consciousness on behavior is secondary. Consciousness does not directly cause most of our actions but instead rationalizes them. In that view, free will plays a minor role, if any. We are machines, we act according to unconscious computations, and conscious thought is a cleverly invented narrative to make excuses for the behavior of the machine.

The epiphenomenon hypothesis of consciousness and the after-the-fact hypothesis are both essentially contrarian views. They violate conventional intuition. In conventional intuition, consciousness has two broad properties. First, we have an awareness, or an understanding, or a vivid description, of ourselves and the world around us. Consciousness takes in information. It is an observer. Second, consciousness can also make choices and control our behavior. It is an actor. In the contrarian views, however, intuition is wrong, introspection is naïve, and consciousness has at best only the first property and not the second. It may be a vivid and distorted description of oneself and the world, but it lacks the ability to make choices and control behavior. It is passive perception rather than active control.

The theory of consciousness proposed in this book, once its implications are thought through, ends up standing on the side of conventional intuition and against the contrarian views. Awareness is an informational model, a description, a picture; but the depiction directly alters the thing that it depicts. It has the capacity to shape the processing in the brain and to control behavior. In an earlier chapter I suggested that awareness was something like the mission statement of a business. It is a description that also makes it so. The attention schema theory allows awareness to serve both as a descriptive model and as a controller, and that double function lies at the philosophical heart of the theory, just as it lies at the heart of the human intuitive understanding of consciousness.

Do we often rationalize our behavior after the fact? Yes. Indeed, one's informational model of oneself contains inherent, inevitable simplifications, just by virtue of being a model. Models are simplifications of the things they represent. Moreover, much of the information in the brain never reaches consciousness. We frequently act without any conscious knowledge why, and then make up false reasons to explain it. Consciousness is hardly the sole controller of behavior. But in the current theory, consciousness is at least one part of the control process.

Consciousness A and Consciousness B

In the attention schema theory, awareness is a model constructed by the social machinery of the brain. Yet there are two flavors to this model. In a sense, the theory describes two related but different types of awareness. One (let us call it awareness type A) is the model we construct and attribute to ourselves. The second (let us call it awareness type B) is the model we construct and attribute to something else, such as when we perceive awareness to be present in another person, in a pet, in a ventriloquist's puppet, or in some other object.

These two types of awareness are by hypothesis similar in their construction, but they have somewhat different dynamics. As discussed in previous chapters, one difference is that the awareness we attribute to others is open-loop (it describes others without directly influencing the thing it describes), whereas the awareness we attribute to ourselves is closed-loop (it describes an inner state but also helps to control that inner state). Despite these differences, the two are related. They are different styles of the same process. When asking whether a particular object has awareness, we are therefore plagued by an ambiguity between awareness A and awareness B. The confusion is not trivial. In real circumstances, people seem to switch back and forth between the two with great ease and without even knowing it.

For example, I had a discussion with a scientific colleague about consciousness. He was arguing against my attention schema theory and said, "A bird doesn't have an STS or a TPJ in its brain. According to you, therefore, a bird should not be conscious. But if you watch a bird getting eaten by a cat, if you watch it struggle and cry out, how can you look at it and deny that it is conscious? Of course it is."

First, as far as my theory goes, a bird might be conscious. I don't know. I don't know if the avian brain computes an attention schema. Since at least some species of bird are highly social, I'd guess that they do compute something like an attention schema, use it to keep track of each other's attentional states, use it to model their own attentional states, and therefore are probably conscious in some sense—even if the bird brain does lack an STS and a TPJ.

But I have a deeper problem with my colleague's argument. His argument conflates consciousness A and consciousness B. When he looks at an animal in distress, because of the strong visual and sound cues, because of the motion of the animal and the intensity of its voice, my colleague's social machinery is engaged. His brain constructs a model of awareness, a model of a conscious mind, a model of emotion and intention, and attributes it to that animal. He constructs consciousness type B and projects it onto the animal. The bird has consciousness type B. I am convinced. My friend has won that point. But whether the bird has consciousness type A, whether it constructs awareness and attributes awareness to itself, is much harder to figure out.

Consider a situation that is all too real. Suppose a loved one is in a coma and the question arises, does the person still have any human awareness, or is she a mental blank? Should life support be removed or not? The family who sits at the bedside may insist that the patient has a conscious mind buried deep inside. They know it. They feel it. It is tangible. Sometimes she looks at them, sometimes she twitches a hand seemingly in reaction, sometimes her face has a look of emotion. The Terri Shiavo case[9] comes to mind. Her parents, observing her movements and facial expressions, were certain of her personhood, her conscious presence. The parents, presumably without knowing it, were reporting consciousness type B: a perceptual model of consciousness that was constructed inside the minds of the family members and attributed to the patient in a coma. It led them to feel, to intuit, to develop a vivid certainty that their loved one was aware. To them her soul was still present.

Her husband, with the backing of the legal system, wanted to end the patient's care, remove the feeding tube, and let her pass away. In his claim, his wife had no mind or consciousness left. There was no possibility of any functioning machinery for the production of consciousness. After seven years of legal wrangling that reached all levels of the legal system and even involved President George W. Bush signing a law specifically to keep her alive, the husband won the case and her life support was withdrawn. Medical evidence after the fact indicated that, with an almost total loss of cortical pyramidal cells, the neurons that allow for communication among cortical regions, she probably had insufficient machinery in her brain for any conscious life. The evidence strongly suggested that she had no consciousness type A. She had no capacity to construct a perceptual model of consciousness and attribute it to herself.

In a sense, the wrenching emotional fight over Terri Schiavo was an unintentional confusion between two meanings, between consciousness B (which Terri had, as attested by her parents) and consciousness A (which, on available evidence, she probably did not have).

I suspect most people, on thinking through this and other similar examples, would conclude that consciousness type B, the consciousness that people attribute to other people, is not real. It is a guess about someone else that might or might not be correct. Consciousness type A, the consciousness that a brain constructs for itself, is the real stuff. In the attention schema theory, however, this common intuition is wrong. Consciousness can be attributed to oneself or to others. Despite the differences in detail and in dynamics, consciousness A and consciousness B are essentially the same material. One is no more or less real than the other.

To get at this idea more clearly I would like to return to an example that I briefly discussed in Chapter 7. This example is less fraught with emotion than a comatose medical case and thus perhaps is easier to dissect intellectually. Consider ventriloquism. Most people think of ventriloquism as an illusion of hearing and seeing. You hear the performer's words and see the puppet's mouth move at the same time, and therefore the sound seems to come from the puppet. But ventriloquism is more than a sensory illusion. The sensory illusion is actually quite incidental. If you watch ventriloquism on TV or on YouTube, the sound comes from the same speaker location anyway, regardless of whether the puppet or the performer is speaking. The visual-capture illusion is the same in both cases—a voice seems to come from a moving mouth, even though the sound is actually coming from a different source—yet you are entranced by the puppet speaking and not by the performer speaking. Why? The charm of ventriloquism really depends on a social illusion. Your brain constructs a model of a conscious mind and attributes it to the puppet.

Ventriloquism is not a cognitive error. You do not mistakenly believe the puppet to be conscious. You know cognitively that there is no brain in the puppet's head. But perceptually, you fall for the illusion. That is what makes ventriloquism fun. You can't help feeling as though awareness were emanating from the puppet as it looks around the room and comments on its surroundings. In fact, your social machinery builds two models of minds, one that you project onto the performer and the other that you project onto the puppet. Ventriloquists have worked out a set of tricks to enhance this illusion of two separate minds. That is why the puppet always has a different tone of voice and usually argues with the performer. At this point in the stage version of my scientific story, I normally reach into a bag and take out Kevin, a hairy two-foot-tall orangutan puppet, and carry on a conversation with him. I try to be polite and stick to the science, but he cracks jokes and offends the audience with comments about my hand up his backside. I am a passable ventriloquist. I am not superb, but it doesn't matter because the social illusion is so powerful that it works anyway. Kevin the orangutan projects his own consciousness and his own distinct personality.

He has consciousness type B.

It seems crazy to insist that the puppet's consciousness is real. And yet, I argue that it is. The puppet's consciousness is a real informational model that is constructed inside the neural machinery of the audience members and the performer. It is assigned a spatial location inside the puppet. The impulse to dismiss the puppet's consciousness derives, I think, from the implicit belief that *real* consciousness is an utterly different quantity, perhaps a ghostly substance, or an emergent state, or an oscillation, or an experience, present inside of a person's head. Given the contrast between a real if ethereal phenomenon inside of a person's head and a mere computed model that somebody has attributed to a puppet, then obviously the puppet isn't really conscious. But in the present theory, all consciousness is a "mere" computed model attributed to an object. That is what consciousness is made out of. One's brain can attribute it to oneself or to something else. Consciousness is an attribution.

Indeed, we might say that the phraseology is at fault. Things don't strictly "have" consciousness, nor "are" they conscious. Instead, informational models of consciousness are constructed in the brain and attributed to objects.

It is difficult to pry oneself away from the idea that consciousness is an intrinsic property of a person. Somehow it is easier to get at the concept when thinking about a property like beauty. We all know that beauty is, proverbially, in the eye of the beholder. Nothing is intrinsically beautiful. Instead, beautiful implies a relationship between the beholder and the beheld. A narcissist might behold beauty in him- or herself (we might call it beauty type A), but just because it is self-beheld does not make it more real. You might behold beauty in someone else (we might call it beauty type B), but just because it is attributed to something outside yourself does not make it less real. Whether you see beauty in yourself or in something else, it is all more or less the same property. Beauty is an attribution.

I admit that the suggestion is counterintuitive. I seem to be saying that a puppet can be conscious. A tree can be conscious. A hunk of rock can be conscious. They can all be conscious in more or less the same sense that a human is conscious. The reason is that, according to the attention schema theory, human consciousness is not quite what we think it is. It is not something a person has, floating inside. It is an attribution. It is a relationship between an attributer and an attributee.

In some ways, to say, "This puppet is conscious," is like saying, "This puppet is orange." We think of color as a property of an object, but technically, this is not so. Orange is not an intrinsic property of my orangutan puppet's fabric. Some set of wavelengths reflects from the cloth, enters your eye, and is processed in your brain. Orange is a construct of the brain. The same set of wavelengths might be perceived as reddish, greenish, or bluish, depending on circum-stances. (For a particularly good set of illusions that demonstrate the subjective quality of color, see the work of Dale Purves displayed on his Web site.[10] See also his book.[11]) To say the puppet is orange is shorthand for saying, "A brain has attributed orange to it." Similarly, according to the present theory, to say that the puppet is conscious is to say, "A brain has attributed consciousness to it." To say that a tree is conscious is to say, "A brain has constructed the informational model of awareness and attributed it to that tree." To say that I myself am conscious is to say, "My own brain has constructed an informa-tional model of awareness and attributed it to my body." These are all similar acts. They all involve a brain attributing awareness to an object.

Awareness and Evolution: What's It Good for?

In the attention schema theory, awareness is a model of attention. It helps track and predict attention. This knowledge is of obvious value. If you understand someone else's attentional state, you can better predict that person's behavior. If you can better predict that person's behavior, then you can choose your actions more effectively, survive more effectively, and pass on genes more effectively. Likewise, if you understand your own attentional state, you can better predict and guide your own behavior. Awareness has an evolutionary advantage. It has a *use*.

I will now take a step in the reasoning that is not legitimate and not correct but is so easy to make that many people may inadver-tently slip in that direction—and I think many people do.

Suppose you attribute awareness to a puppet, or a tree, or an imag-ined ghost. In that case, the awareness is misapplied. If awareness is a model of attention, and attention is a property of a brain, then attrib-uting awareness to a thing that has no brain is a misuse of the skill. Its advantage is negated. In this view, attributing awareness to an object with no brain is an evolutionary mistake. It is counterproductive. No frivolous imagination allowed! Consciousness should not be attributed to puppets! Or trees! Or "angry" storms! Or ghosts! Only to actual biological beings with complex brains. Anything else is an error, a drain on the human endeavor, an evolutionary hindrance. This perspective dismisses the ghosts and the gods and the spirits with a dose of hard-nosed pragmatism. It is, I find, a common position among scientists with whom I discuss the topic.

The difficulty with this pragmatic perspective lies in assuming that any trait has an evolutionary purpose. There really is no such thing as an evolutionary purpose. Traits evolve and once present can be used in a great variety of contexts, some that have nothing to do with the original evolutionary path. This reinvention of adaptive uses was first suggested by Darwin.[12] Steven Jay Gould elaborated on the idea.[13,14] He called it "cooption," or "exaptation," when a trait that evolved for one adaptive function is taken over at a later time by a different function. He pointed out that some traits evolve for no good adaptive advantage of their own, much as spandrels, the non-functional empty spaces here and there in buildings, arise because of other surrounding architectural necessities.[15] These spandrel-like traits, which have no obvious original function, can eventually take on an adaptive function. Evolution works opportunistically. There is, of course, no moral imperative and no adaptive advantage in us humans trying to stay true to what we imagine to be the evolutionary purpose of a trait.

As an example of the multiple functions of a biological trait, take the case of the human foot. It evolved in a way that makes it good for walking and running. But is the purpose of a foot to help us walk and run? If I use my foot for some other reason, am I violating an evolutionary purpose? Am I guilty of a transgression? Hardly. People use feet in a great variety of opportunistic ways. We tap rhythms, we kick each other, we use our feet to showcase fashionable shoes, we tickle a child's feet as a part of social interaction. These uses have nothing to do with walking or running. A foot doesn't really have a *purpose*, in the sense of a particular, proper, sanctioned way that it is intended to be deployed. Instead it has many uses—some more common, some less common, some for which it is better fitted, some for which it is less well fitted, some that provide an adaptive advantage, and some that might not.

The same flexibility applies to the trait of consciousness, just as it does to any other evolved trait. Throughout this book I've proposed that awareness evolved as a predictive model of attention. Supposing this hypothesis is correct, it in no way implies that awareness is limited to that particular function. Awareness may have a great range of uses. Evolution may have shaped it further such that it contributes to many behavioral functions.

Once we see consciousness as linked to social perception, once we understand that one's own awareness and one's perception of awareness in others are manifestations of the same underlying process, then we have a vast range of new possible adaptive uses to which consciousness can be put.

Consciousness, for example, could be used as a tool for social cohesion. If you perceive consciousness in someone, then you empathize and you cooperate. If you perceive consciousness in an object, a talisman, then maybe you create a cultural focus, an item around which the community can bond. If you can generate a model of consciousness for a person who is described to you, who is in your imagination, who is not actually present, then maybe you can maintain social bonds across distances when messages are carried from person to person. When the members of an audience listen to a story and invest themselves in the larger-than-life fictional characters of the story, perceiving mind and soul in those characters, then the audience becomes knitted together by a common mythology. In all of these contexts, the adaptive advantage of consciousness, of perceiving it in others and perceiving it in oneself, has more to do with being human and relating to other humans, with being part of a community, with enhancing human effectiveness through cohesion, than it does with the specific task of predicting attentional state.

The idea that consciousness plays a role in social cohesion has been suggested by others.[16–18] I believe the idea is plausible and fully consistent with the attention schema theory. The attention schema theory explains the possible starting point, the specific mechanism, the pragmatic, first-order survival advantage to awareness—a predictive model of attention. But a trait that has such a pervasive effect on behavior surely must serve many uses. If something as mechanical and straight-forward as a foot can have half a dozen common uses beyond the obvious use in locomotion, then awareness must surely be put to a range of uses beyond tracking and predicting attentional state.

Fins evolved to help fish swim. Yet they can also be used to drag a body across the ground. Hence, incrementally, the legs of tetrapods evolved during the Devonian period. Legs evolved to help animals walk. Yet the front legs, when spread out with sufficient surface area, can catch the air. Hence wings evolved. Perhaps, as proposed in this book, awareness evolved as a predictive model of attention— specific, useful, limited. Here I suggest that a predictive model of attention is unlikely to be the only functional use of this trait of awareness. Instead, in humans, awareness may have evolved into our social and humanistic wings. We are the most social of all species on earth, in the sense that we have the most complex social universe. We spend our lives embedded in a social matrix. One recent suggestion, for example, is that awareness serves the adaptive function of making life emotionally lovely and therefore worth living.[19]

Consider human spirituality—the tendency to see spirits everywhere, to see mind not only in ourselves and in each other, not only in pets and other animals, but also in cars that we get mad at when they don't start; in house plants that we talk to as we water them; in the favorite stuffed animals of children, like Hobbes of Calvin and Hobbes; in storms that seem like the products of angry spirits; in the empty spaces at night when you get the creepy irrational feeling that someone is in your house uninvited. It is really only a small step from the universal perception of mind everywhere to the more formalized notions of ghosts, angels, devils, and deities. However much the nonsuperstitious may smile at the superstitious, we are all engaged in more or less the same habit: actively constructing a perceptual world suffused with spirit. We are all spiritual. Let me make sure the statement is unambiguous: even the atheistic scientists among us, such as myself, cannot help being spiritual. It is built into our social machinery. It is what people are.

One might ask, what could possibly be the adaptive advantage of so much misapplied social perception? Granted, perceiving mind in ourselves, and perceiving mind in other people and in animals, has its uses. It is good for behavioral prediction. But really, what is the adaptive advantage of perceiving mind in things that have no brains? Why so much irrationality?

Why spirituality? This question is the target of an enormous amount of theorizing.[1-5] One common proposal is that spirituality must have some definite benefit to people. Since we humans have it, and have it like crazy in every culture, it must somehow be good for us, otherwise the trait would have died out. Perhaps religious mythology binds together a community. Group cohesion can help the individuals in the group survive. Hence spirituality offers a survival advantage. Or perhaps spirituality helps people feel more socially connected and thus helps in psychological health. In 2001, reviewing the large literature on religion and health, Koenig and Cohen[20] reported that seventy-nine percent of the studies obtained a positive link. Religiosity was linked to better health. This type of finding makes headlines and is all too easy to politicize. The argument has been made that merely being in a social group of any type, religious or not, provides the health benefit.[21]

Another hypothesis to explain spirituality suggests that it does not itself benefit us but is a side product of something else beneficial. It is an evolutionary spandrel, or an exaptation.[13] One of the most important proposals in this literature is Barrett's[3] suggestion that people have a hyperactive agency detection device (HADD). In this hypothesis the human brain contains machinery for detecting agency, such as detecting a predator that might be sneaking up on you. It is advantageous to tune that detector to a state of hyperactivity. It is better to be jumpy, to detect agency where it does not exist and remain safe than to make the opposite error and get eaten. Because of the hyperactivity of this device, humans are prone to believe in spirits and ghosts. The cost is smaller than the benefit.

While I appreciate the idea of the HADD, I suggest that the advantage of our human hypersociality goes way beyond the detection of predators. Our greatest survival advantage lies in our incredible social networking, our ability to instantly intuit other people's mind states, our ability to construct rich and complex models of each other, to construct a web of communication that proceeds under the surface of language and that gives each word in spoken language a halo of extra meaning. Think of the power of the Internet and the power of social media. Think of how each advance in group communication fundamentally alters our world. Human social intelligence was evolution's invention of the equivalent of the Internet. If one consequence of this incredible skill set is a little superstition on the side, so be it. The benefit far outweighs the cost. Tuning down the intensity of human social perception, making us less hypersocial in order to reduce our spiritual misattributions, would be an extremely counteradaptive adjustment.

It is a bit like the cost–benefit ratio of wearing clothes. On the up side, clothes protect us from the elements. On the down side, they add a small amount of weight that we must carry around, thereby wasting energy. The cost is rather absurdly negligible compared to the enormous benefit. Just so, I would suggest that the cost to humans of being hypersocial, of having social machinery so constantly active, so tuned to a hair trigger, so revved, that we tend to see mind all around us, even in things that don't have brains—the cost of that condition is actually quite small compared to the enormous, fundamental, humanity-defining benefit. We would be nothing without our sociality.

To me personally, the most reasonable approach to spirituality is to accept two simultaneous truths. One, literally and objectively, there is no spirit world. Minds do not float independently of bodies and brains. Two, perceptually, there is a spirit world. We live in a perceptual world, a world simulated by the brain, in which consciousness inhabits many things around us, including sometimes empty space. In the same way, most of us are comfortable knowing that, literally and objectively, white is a muddy mixture of all wavelengths and has no purity whatsoever, whereas perceptually, white is pure luminance without any color. We do not mind the contradiction because we understand where it comes from. The perceptual world and the objective world do not always match. We sometimes must live with both sets of knowledge. Neither side can be ignored. We cannot help living in the world that our perceptual machinery constructs for us, but it is also useful to know as much as we can about the literal, objective world.

The Consciousness of Nonhuman Animals

Are nonhuman animals aware? Once again, I do not know the answer to this question. But I can apply the attention schema theory and see what answer the theory gives.

We can certainly construct models of conscious minds and attribute them to nonhuman animals. People are generally quite certain that their pets are conscious. Just look at them. See how they act. Look at the expression on Fifi's face. Isn't it obvious? This certainty is the result of informational models of consciousness constructed in the human brain and attributed to the pets. Animals have consciousness type B, to use the terminology of the previous sections. We attribute consciousness to them.

But one can ask a deeper question: do nonhuman animals have the neuronal machinery to construct informational models of consciousness and attribute them to others? Can a cat attribute consciousness to me? Can a dog attribute consciousness to another dog? Can a horse attribute consciousness to itself? Do animals have consciousness type A?

At least some level of social perception is probably widespread in the animal kingdom. Few species have a full-blown, human-like ability for reading other creatures' minds with great subtlety, though the question of theory of mind in nonhuman animals is still in debate.[22-26]

In the present theory, awareness does not depend on social perception in general but instead on one specific aspect of it, the reconstruction of attention. In this hypothesis, any animal that can construct a rich model of another's attentional state knows what awareness is; and any animal that maintains a model of its own attentional state is aware. Whether a particular species has these abilities is an empirical question, but the bar is lower than for advanced social cognition. Humans may (or may not) have the most complex and sophisticated social intelligence on earth, but other animals should have awareness.

Without direct empirical evidence on how animals construct models of attention, it is hard to know which animals might be conscious according to the present theory. If I had to hazard a guess, I would say that most mammals and most birds probably construct something like awareness as we understand it. They almost certainly have attentional processes similar to ours and therefore could make use of an attention schema. In one study, an analysis of the way dogs play with each other suggested that they have an acute perception of each other's state of attention.[24] When dog A sends a signal to engage dog B in play, dog A seems to evaluate the direction and extent of dog B's attention. If dog B's attention is already directed at dog A, then dog A employs a subtle gesture, maybe a wiggle or a look. If dog B's attention is directed away from dog A, then dog A employs a more forceful gesture to engage dog B, maybe a bark. This observation, neatly documented, may seem like a demonstration of the obvious, at least to any dog owner. But it is particularly interesting in the present discussion because it directly tests the ability of dogs to construct a model or schema of another dog's attention. If the attention schema theory is correct, then this observation by itself indicates that dogs probably have awareness.

I have less of a sense of the possibilities in nonmammalian and nonavian animals. I do not know of any studies testing whether lizards use the data-handling method of attention as it is understood in mammals or construct models of attentional state.

One of the least intuitive implications of the present theory is that awareness is a specialized, quirky, limited faculty, a weird product of evolution, not a measure of general intelligence. Super-intelligent aliens from outer space, if such things exist, might have cities and technologies and yet lack anything like sentience. In the same way, they might lack fingers, or ears, or a spleen. If we met them, however, and if they behaved in complex and intelligent ways, we would probably attribute consciousness to them. They would have consciousness B, meaning that we would be able to perceive consciousness in them. We might have an intuitive impression of consciousness in them or convince ourselves that they have it. We might treat them as though they do. But to know whether they have consciousness A, whether they have an ability to construct informational models of awareness and attribute those models to others and to themselves, we would have to do neurophysiology experiments on them and study their machinery for social perception and for attention. We would have to figure out whether the alien brain supports the process of attention and contains an attention schema. If so, then by the present theory, that alien brain would be conscious.

Computer Consciousness

While I am on the subject of the consciousness of space aliens, I might as well turn to another favorite topic of the science fiction crowd: the consciousness of computers.

Turing, in his famous paper from 1950,[27] asked whether a computing machine can think. That paper has tended to be interpreted selectively over the years, and therefore it is worth summarizing the original remarkable version here. Turing never asks about awareness or consciousness. He asks whether a computer can think like a human. He proposes a game that involves three human players who communicate only by typed words. Each person has a specific goal. Person 1 tries to guess the gender of the other two, person 2 tries to communicate his or her gender accurately to the guesser, and person 3 is a deceiver who tries anything to mislead the guesser. All three are locked in an intensive game of social intelligence. If you replace the deceiver with a computing machine, will the machine be able to win as often as a real person? If so, then the machine passes a specific, testable, and rather impressive criterion for human-like thinking. In retrospect, Turing's test fits wonderfully with the approach that I take in this book. To Turing, the criterion for human-like thinking is the ability to hold your own in a game of intensive social interaction.

The "Turing test" as it has since developed in popular culture is generally a warped and simplified version of Turing's original idea. In the standard Turing test, you have a conversation with a computer. If you can't tell that it is a computer, and you think that it is an actual conscious human, then the computer passes the Turing test. Curiously, the Turing test is a test for consciousness type B. It is a test for whether you can attribute consciousness to it, not for whether it can attribute consciousness to itself. The Turing test, as it has been reinvented over the years, is less interesting than Turing's original idea.

But can a computer have consciousness type A? Can it construct its own awareness?

In science fiction, when computers become complicated enough or amass enough information, they become conscious. This is the case according to well-known scientific scholars on consciousness such as Isaac Asimov and Arthur C. Clarke. Hal from the movie *2001* comes to mind. So does the machine world from the *Terminator* series, and the malevolent computers of *The Matrix*. Exactly why complexity itself, or increased information storage, or an increase in some other standard computer attribute, would eventually result in awareness is not clear. Computers are already extremely complex. The amount of memory in a supercomputer already rivals that of a human brain. The speed of computation is much greater for a computer than for a human. The Internet links so much information that it vastly exceeds the total amount of information at any one time in normal human consciousness. If consciousness is simply an inevitable result of "enough" complexity or "enough" information, then the prospects do not look bright for reaching enough. It hasn't happened yet. It seems that awareness is not simply more of the same stuff that computers already have. Instead, it is a specific feature that has not yet been programmed into a computer.

According to the attention schema theory, to make a computer aware in the human-like sense, to give it consciousness type A, requires three things. First, the computer must sort its information and control its behavior using the method of attention. It needs to select and enhance signals with the same dynamics that a human does.

Second, the computer must have programmed into it an attention schema to track, simulate, and predict that process of attention. The computer's attention schema must have the idiosyncratic properties of the human attention schema. It cannot be a computer scientist's version, or an engineer's version, an optimized or accurate log of the attentional state. Instead, it needs the metaphorical layer present in the human attention schema. It needs to depict attention as an ethereal substance with a general location in space, as an intelligence that experiences information, as an ectoplasmic force that can flow and cause actions.

Third, the computer needs to be able to link its attention schema (A) to other information, including information on itself (S) and information on the item (X) to which it is directing attention.

For it to be aware of information X, it must be able to construct the larger chunk of information $S + A + X$.

The computer would then be in a position to access that larger representation, read the information therein, summarize it, and report: X comes with awareness, with conscious *experience*, attached to it, and I myself in particular am the one who is aware. When asked about what awareness "feels" like, the computer would again access that model and obtain an answer. It would provide a human-like answer because the information set on which it bases that answer would be similar to the information set on which we humans base our answer.

The attention schema theory therefore gives a specific prescription, a direction for engineers to follow in building a conscious computer.

Given that Deep Blue was programmed to win at chess and that Watson was programmed to win at Jeopardy, I am certain a computer system could be designed and programmed to construct a rich, complex model of attentional state. A computer that can attribute consciousness to others and to itself should be possible. My guess is that by combining the technologies that already exist, and by working along the lines indicated by the attention schema theory, a team of dedicated people with good funding should be able to build an uncannily human-like consciousness within about a decade. If the project is not tackled with quite as much energy or funding as Deep Blue or Watson, then I'm sure it will take longer than a decade. But I consider the outcome to be not only possible but inevitable. We will build computers that can construct their own awareness in the same way that the human brain does.

Conscious computers would have the same usefulness as conscious humans. They would be easier for humans to interact with. Since we are exquisitely good at social interaction, since we tend to think and operate through our social intelligence, a socially intelligent computer, a computer with consciousness that could join the network of minds around it, would make for an effective SUI (social user interface).

Judging once again from popular novels and movies, the science fiction crowd may tend to envision a conscious computer as a machine that can deceive, manipulate, cause sociopolitical cataclysm, take over the world, and generally kill off humanity. None of these properties are desirable. I suggest, however, that megalomania and villainy have nothing to do with the question of consciousness. A dangerous marauding computer could exist perfectly well without awareness. And an aware computer could be a useful tool, just as modern computers are, without malevolently choosing on its own to kill off anything.

Can Consciousness Survive the Death of the Brain?

What does the present theory imply about life after death?

The theory certainly has no room for a spirit that floats free of the body. Consciousness depends on a brain or some other computer constructing it. When the computer goes down, the computations cease. There is one common way, however, in which our conscious minds effectively survive the death of the brain.

Imagine editing a document on a computer. That document file is data on a software platform on the hardware platform of the computer. Suppose you copy the file to a memory stick. Then the computer crashes. The hard drive breaks catastrophically and irreparably. Since you saved your work, you don't mind very much. You put the memory stick in another computer, copy the file, and return to work. You never stop to worry that, strictly speaking, it is not the same file. The old file has died. What you now have is a copy. Since all the important information has been transferred, you are satisfied.

In the attention schema theory, the social machinery in my brain constructs an informational model of a conscious mind, a quirky, idiosyncratic model that is my understanding of myself and my attentive relationship to the rest of the world. $S + A +$ World. The property of awareness is a part of that informational model. The model is what I call my conscious mind. It is information constructed and manipulated on neuronal circuitry. Can that file be copied from my brain to a similar device and run?

Not at high fidelity. I lack a data port in my head and therefore, alas, have no way to copy the information in any detail. But I can make a rough copy. I can spend time with a friend. If I spend enough time and my friend gets to know me well, then he will construct a model in his own brain, an informational model of a mind filled with the quirks and idiosyncracies that reflect me. His model of my mind will be the same general type of data run in the same general manner on the same general hardware architecture as my own conscious mind. It will be a copy, at low resolution, of my consciousness. In effect, I will have been copied over from one computer to another.

I have in my brain a rich, detailed, working model of my grandmother, who has been dead for twenty years now. I can run that model and imagine her voice, her body language, her probable reactions in this or that situation, her emotional tone. She comes to life again in my inner experience. That informational model of a mind, run in my brain, is a low-resolution copy of the model that existed in her brain and that she considered to be her consciousness.

It is trite to say that we live on in the people who remember us. But the theory of consciousness described in this book suggests that there is some literal truth to the idea. Fuzzy copies of our conscious minds exist in all the people who knew us.

This realization leads to an interesting irony. The materialistic view, in which the brain constructs consciousness, is generally considered to be a bleak one without an afterlife. Death is the end. When the brain stops functioning the mind blinks out. The religious find that prospect horrifying and the atheistic have reconciled themselves to it. Some people may even feel comfort that no more experiences, pleasant or unpleasant or just plain tiring, are in the offing after death. I suppose Shakespeare's Hamlet in his "To be or not to be" speech is the most famous case of hoping that nothing too awful comes after death. "For in that sleep of death, what dreams may come, when we have shuffled off this mortal coil…"

If consciousness is information, if it is a vast informational model instantiated on the hardware of the brain, then it actually can survive the death of the body. Information is in principle possible to move from device to device. The irony is that the materialistic view makes mental survival beyond death much more likely, rather than less likely. Far from grinding its heal on the prospect of existence after death, the attention schema theory, an entirely materialistic theory, suggests that the mind's survival after the body's death already happens in a perfectly ordinary way. We get to know each other. We build models of each other. Information is transferred from brain to brain via language and observation.

In theory we can do even better. I consider it a technological inevitability that information will, some day, be scannable directly from the brain and transferrable directly into computers. As embarrassingly sci-fi as that sounds, no theoretical reason stands against it. If the attention schema theory is correct, then human consciousness is information processed in a specific manner. Don't want to die? Download your consciousness onto a central server and live in a simulated world with all the other downloaded souls. When your body dies, the copy of your mind will persist. You need not know the difference. If the simulation is good, you should feel as though you are in a realistic universe. You can possess what seems to be a human body and can walk and live and eat and sleep on the familiar Earth, all simulated, all in the form of information manipulated on computer hardware. At the rate technology is advancing, give it a few centuries. (Alas, I'll be gone by then.)

One of the more intriguing possibilities is simulating a world of one's own design. The physics and appearance of the simulated world need not match the real world. Are you obsessed by Harry Potter? Then live in a world where Potter-style magic is possible and you can learn to harness it by attending a school for witchcraft and wizardry. Wish you could live in Middle Earth? Then do so. Train as a Jedi?

Why not? Want to get blue and live on Pandora? Go ahead. A Star Trek fanatic? Then live in a universe where the Starship Enterprise actually exists and can actually travel at warp speed. Want diversity? Open a door and move from one invented reality to the other.

You could even park your simulated self in front of a simulated monitor in your simulated universe and have a Skype chat with the people on the outside, the people in the real world who are not dead yet, who have not yet chosen to download their information. People could talk daily to their dead relatives, provided the relatives have the time to spare among the many amusements of their simulated playground. Or, more mind-bendingly, the simulated you could have a chat with the biological you on the outside, the original you who decided to download your mind mid-way through your life.

As long as the computer hardware persists, as long as someone or something on the outside maintains it, there is no particular reason for you to die in the simulated world. And never mind people on the outside sustaining the hardware. Build a sturdy, self-sustaining computer architecture, build it deep underground where it can be protected, where geothermal energy could provide it with a thin trickle of energy to keep it going and how long could it last? You could be ageless and immune to all disease or disability. A limited lifespan could be programmed into the simulation, if necessary, to avoid hitting limits on computing resources. But theoretically one could continue indefinitely in a simulated body in a simulated world, as a conscious being experiencing a simulated life.

I'm not quite sure if such an existence is better described as heaven or hell. It depends on the simulated world, I suppose. Either way, the technology is theoretically possible and in my view, as I noted before, inevitable. We humans are expert at inventing ways to entertain ourselves and make ourselves comfortable.

It has been said that people invented God. People will invent the afterlife too.

At this point in the discussion a sneaking suspicion comes to mind, described by Bostrum in 2003.[28] What if our current reality is exactly such a simulation? Maybe a complex simulated universe has already been created by computer scientists in some meta-universe that we don't know about. When our own computer scientists create a plausible simulated reality, maybe that will be a simulation within a simulation.

Now my head starts to hurt. I don't *think* we live in an artificially constructed simulation. But I admit I have no basis for knowing. It is, at least, theoretically possible.

Does God Exist?

I might as well go for the big question. The God debate between science and religion can be incendiary. I detect on both sides a tendency to start with a conclusion and then to erect the reasons. I don't like that approach, especially on the scientific side, because it cheapens the intellectual arguments. Here I would like to avoid the trap of partisanship. My goal is narrowly defined: what does the present theory of consciousness say about the existence of deities?

A common argument against the existence of a deity takes the following form: science has a natural explanation for thing X. Therefore, we do not need a supernatural explanation. Therefore, we do not need a deity. The most obvious example of this argument invokes Darwinian natural selection. We have a natural explanation for the diversity of life on Earth. Therefore, we do not need a supernatural explanation. Therefore, we do not need God. Richard Dawkins' book, *The God Delusion*,[29] comes to mind as one of many, many examples of this type of argument.

The origin of the universe also frequently enters the debate. If physicists have a scientific theory of the origin of the universe, then we do not need a supernatural explanation and thus do not need a deity. Stephen Hawking's book, *The Grand Design*,[30] explores this argument. As pointed out by many scholars, physicists actually have yet to devise a workable, self-contained theory, accepted by the scientific consensus, that explains the existence of the universe. In the minds of many people, therefore, God still has some wiggle room.

All of the arguments noted above focus on what a deity might or might not do, what it might or might not have created in the past. These common and endless arguments, however, avoid the central issue of what a deity is supposed to *be*. What is a god made out of? Can that stuff exist? Is a god even possible?

Across all cultures and all religions, universally, people consider God to be a conscious mind. God is aware. God consciously chooses to make things happen. In physical reality the tree fell, the storm bowled over the house, the man survived the car crash, the woman died prematurely, the earth orbits the sun, the cosmos exists. For many people these events, big and small, must have a consciousness and an intentionality behind them. God is that consciousness.

Without consciousness, the God concept becomes meaningless. If God is a nonconscious complex process that can create patterns and direct the affairs of the universe, then God obviously and trivially exists. The physical universe itself fits that description. The critical question is whether consciousness lies behind the events of the universe. If so, then God exists. If not, then God does not exist.

Armed with a theory of what consciousness is and how it is constructed, we can directly address the God question. Are the events in the universe associated with an awareness? If yes, then God. If no, then no God.

According to the attention schema theory, consciousness is information. It is information of a specific type constructed in the brain. It is a quirky, weird product of evolution, like wings, or like eyebrows, or like navels. It is constructed by a brain and attributed to something. Like beauty, another construct of the brain, consciousness is in the eye of the beholder. A brain can behold consciousness in others (consciousness type B as I have called it) or behold consciousness in itself (consciousness type A as I have called it). These two types of consciousness have clear differences but are essentially two flavors of the same thing.

The universe has consciousness type B. That consciousness is an informational model constructed in the brains of many (though not all) people and attributed to the collection of all events that are otherwise inexplicable. The cosmos is conscious in much the same way that anything else is. Its consciousness is made of the same stuff as our own consciousness—information instantiated in the hardware platform of the brain. The universe is conscious in the same sense that it is beautiful. It is conscious because brains attribute consciousness to it, and that is the only way that anything is ever conscious.

The universe almost certainly lacks consciousness type A. It lacks any mechanism to construct its own informational models of minds and attribute them to others or to itself.

Does God exist?

In the attention schema theory the question is moot. Or at least, the answer is more no than yes, but not entirely one or the other. In the present theory of consciousness, no conscious intentionality preceded the universe. Consciousness is a construct of the brain and thus emerged only with the evolution of the brain. Consciousness is probably only a few hundred million years old at most, in a universe that is, by the latest estimate I've heard, about 13.75 billion years old. There is no God of a traditional form, no being made of pure thought or will or spirit that created the universe. Consciousness cannot exist without a hardware system to support the computations. Consciousness by itself does not have the physical capability to move or create matter. That's not what consciousness is. Most people would consider this description to be strictly atheistic. And it is.

And yet there is another side to the story. According to the theory, the statement "X is conscious" means "a brain (or other computational device) constructed an informational model of consciousness and attributed it to X." In this theory, a universal, deistic consciousness does actually exist. It is as real as any other consciousness. If brains attribute consciousness to X, then X is conscious, in the only way that anything is conscious. If we can say the universe is beautiful and find no difficulty with that claim, even knowing that it is beautiful only as a result of intelligent, emotional, and aesthetic beings perceiving it that way, even knowing that before any complex beings existed the beauty of the universe was undefined, then likewise, the universe has an encompassing God-style consciousness, and it does so as a result of intelligent biological beings constructing it that way, because all consciousness is attribution.

The attention schema theory may possibly be the only known scientific theory that is both atheistic and deistic.

My point in this theological section is not to try to twist science until it can justify religion. I am not attempting to shore up deistic thinking. I am also not trying to knock down religion. In the context of this book at least, I have no social or political agenda. The brain is what it is; people are the biological things we are. My interest here is narrowly scientific. The attention schema theory is my best scientific attempt to understand the biological phenomenon of consciousness. When I try to put aside the rationalizations, spin, agendas, and culture wars, when I try to apply the theory to some of the deepest human questions, questions about philosophy and culture and religion, the resulting answers are weird and fit no expected form. They do not entirely vindicate either side of the standard debates. They disturb everyone all around. The conscious mind is a mechanistic computation but it also has a type of free will. The spirit world exists but only as information instantiated on the hardware of the brain. It has a perceptual reality that is hard to ignore, if not a literal reality. In the same way, the deistic consciousness does and doesn't exist. A ventriloquist puppet is and isn't conscious. Spirits are and aren't present. Consciousness can and can't survive the death of the body.

The strangeness and nuance of the answers should not be surprising. The standard questions were formulated long ago from a position of relative human ignorance. They were formulated without any specific theory of brain or consciousness. The age-old questions are simply not well aligned to a theory in which consciousness is an attribution instead of a possession.

18

Explaining the Magic Trick

At the beginning of this book I described a little boy who was trying to explain an amazing magic trick to his father.

The boy's explanation?

"It's easy. The magician makes it happen."

The explanation, of course, explains nothing. To the uncritical mind it might sound good, but it contains an oh-so-minor gap in the logic. The same nonexplanatory explanation could stand in for almost every attempt to date to explain consciousness. Whether scientific, philosophical, or theological, theories of consciousness tend to point to a magician rather than construct an explanation.

What causes consciousness? According to Hippocrates and every neuroscientist since, the brain does. That is probably true, but is not an explanation. According to Descartes, it is a magic fluid in the brain. According to Kant, it is divinely supplied. It is something he called an "a priori form," a term he seemed to use as a euphemism for "inexplicably present." According to various modern theories, it is caused by a vibration or oscillation in neuronal activity. Or it is caused by feedback of information from higher to lower areas in the brain. Or it is caused by complexity. Or it is caused by the massive integration of information in the brain. Throughout this book, I've noted and described about thirty hypotheses or variants of hypotheses. Many more hypotheses exist. Yet most of them share an inconvenient attribute. In each case, they point to a magician. Exactly how you get from the particular magician to the property of awareness, by what logic awareness itself occurs, remains obscure. Theories of consciousness tend to contain, buried in them somewhere, a gap in the logic between the proposed mechanism and the magic.

It seems fair at this point to evaluate whether the attention schema theory contains the same gap. Does it merely point to a magician, or does it provide a possible explanation?

Note that two distinct questions can be asked about the theory. One is whether the theory is *correct*. That is a tall order. No scientist should stand under the mission accomplished sign. I think the theory is *plausible*. I think it is logical. I think it aligns with a great deal of existing data. I am enthusiastic about it and grateful to have had the chance to lay it out in this book. But only future experiments, probably a great diversity of them over many decades, can convince the scientific community.

A second question, easier to answer, is whether the theory provides any explanation at all, or whether it leaves the traditional gap between the mechanism and awareness itself.

Obviously, I believe the theory provides an explanation.

In the attention schema theory, awareness is information. Not only are we aware *of* information, but the awareness itself *is* information. It is specific information computed by a specific system in the brain.

When a data-processing device such as the brain introspects, that is to say consults internal data, and on that basis concludes, assigns a high degree of certainty to the conclusion, and reports that it has physically unexplainable magic inside of it, the simplest scientific explanation is that its information is not precisely accurate. That information may be useful. It may provide a quick sketch of something real that is helpful to monitor. But the sketch is not precisely accurate. That internal data set describes an experienceness, an inner feeling, a mind apprehending sensations and emotions and ideas. The data set describes an awareness like energy or plasma, invisible and yet palpable. The machine, relying on its inner data, concludes that it experiences the blueness of blue, or the coldness of cold, the intensity of joy, the X-ness of X. It concludes that a real awareness is present, and it assigns a high degree of certainty to the conclusion. It can't help that conclusion because the data available to it provide that information.

Nothing in the brain's internal data describes awareness as a mere informational description, or as a construct of neuronal circuits. Nothing in the data set describes the actuality. Hence, when asked, the machine (once again relying on its inner data) concludes that awareness is not mere information, not a mere construct of circuits, but is an actual presence.

The theory is truly explanatory in the sense that it explains the observables. It explains how an information-processing machine can scan its internal data and so find, discover, conclude, decide, assign certainty that it is aware, that it is aware of this or that, that awareness has all the properties that humans normally ascribe to it. The theory explains how a brain can decide with such confidence that it has an inner experience. It explains how a brain can attribute that particular, complex, rich, idiosyncratic combination of properties to itself, to others, to pets, and even to ghosts and to gods.

Notes

Chapter 1: The Magic Trick

1. Gross, C.G. (1999). *Brain, Vision, Memory: Tales in the History of Neuroscience.* Cambridge, MA: Bradford Books, MIT Press.

2. Descartes, R. (1641). Meditations on first philosophy. In *The Philosophical Writings of René Descartes.* Translated by J. Cottingham, R. Stoothoff, and D. Murdoch. Cambridge, UK: Cambridge University Press.

3. Kant, E. (1781). *Critique of Pure Reason.* Translated by J. M. D. Meiklejohn, Project Gutenberg. Retrieved January 22, 2013, from http://www.gutenberg.org/ebooks/4280.

4. Crick, F., and Koch, C. (1990). Toward a neurobiological theory of consciousness. *Semin. Neurosci.* 2: 263–275.

5. Fries, P. (2009). Neuronal gamma-band synchronization as a fundamental process in cortical computation. *Annu. Rev. Neurosci.* 32: 209–224.

6. Palva, S., and Palva, J.M. (2007). New vistas for alpha-frequency band oscillations. *Trends Neurosci.* 30: 150–158.

7. Schroeder, C.E., Wilson, D.A., Radman, T., Scharfman, H., and Lakatos, P. (2010). Dynamics of active sensing and perceptual selection. *Curr. Opin. Neurobiol.* 20: 172–176.

8. Chalmers, D. (1995). Facing up to the problem of consciousness. *J. Conscious. Stud.* 2: 200–219.

9. Bowler, P.J. (2003). *Evolution: The History of an Idea* (3rd ed.). Berkeley: University of California Press.

10. Darwin, C. (1859). *On the Origin of Species by Means of Natural Selection.* London: John Murray Press.

11. Linnaeus, C. (1758). System of nature through the three kingdoms of nature, according to classes, orders, genera and species, with characters, differences, synonyms, places. Stockholm: L. Salvius.

12. Huxley, L. (1900). *The Life and Letters of Thomas Henry Huxley.* London: Macmillan.

13. Graziano, M.S.A. (2008). *The Intelligent Movement Machine: An Ethological Perspective on the Primate Motor System.* Oxford, UK: Oxford University Press

14. Graziano, M.S.A. (2010). *God, Soul, Mind, Brain: A Neuroscientist's Reflections on the Spirit World.* Teaticket MA: Leapfrog Press.

15. Graziano, M.S.A., and Kastner, S. (2011). Human consciousness and its relationship to social neuroscience: a novel hypothesis. *Cogn. Neurosci.* 2: 98–113.

Chapter 2: Introducing the Theory

1. Karnath, H.O., Ferber, S., and Himmelbach, M. (2001). Spatial awareness is a function of the temporal not the posterior parietal lobe. *Nature* 411: 950–953.

2. Vallar, G., and Perani, D. (1986). The anatomy of unilateral neglect after right-hemisphere stroke lesions. A clinical/CT-scan correlation study in man. *Neuropsychologia* 24: 609–622.

3. Graziano, M.S.A. (2010). *God, Soul, Mind, Brain: A Neuroscientist's Reflections on the Spirit World.* Teaticket, MA: Leapfrog Press.

4. Graziano, M.S.A., and Kastner, S. (2011). Human consciousness and its relationship to social neuroscience: A novel hypothesis. *Cogn. Neurosci.* 2: 98–113.

5. Treisman, A., and Gelade, G. (1980). A feature-integration theory of attention. *Cogn. Psychol.* 12: 97–136.

6. Beck, D.M., and Kastner, S. (2009). Top-down and bottom-up mechanisms in biasing competition in the human brain. *Vision Res.* 49: 1154–1165.

7. Desimone, R., and Duncan, J. (1995). Neural mechanisms of selective visual attention. *Annu. Rev. Neurosci.* 18: 193–222.

8. Moore, T., Armstrong, K., and Fallah, M. (2003). Visuomotor origins of covert spatial attention. *Neuron* 40: 671–683.

9. Selfridge, O.G. (1959). Pandemonium: a paradigm for learning. In D.V. Blake and A.M. Uttley (Eds.), *Mechanistic Thought Processes*. London: H.M. Stationary Office, pp. 511–529.

10. Koch, C., and Tsuchiya, N. (2007). Attention and consciousness: two distinct brain processes. *Trends Cogn. Sci.* 11: 16–22.

11. Lamme, V.A. (2004). Separate neural definitions of visual consciousness and visual attention: A case for phenomenal awareness. *Neural Netw.* 17: 861–872.

12. O'Regan, J.K., and Noë, A. (2001). A sensorimotor account of vision and visual consciousness. *Behav. Brain Sci.* 24: 939–973.

13. Posner, M.I. (1994). Attention: the mechanisms of consciousness. *Proc. Natl. Acad. Sci. U. S. A.* 91: 7398–7403.

14. Kentridge, R.W., Heywood, C.A., and Weiskrantz, L. (2004). Spatial attention speeds discrimination without awareness in blindsight. *Neuropsychologia* 42: 831–835.

15. Naccache, L., Blandin, E., and Dehaene, S. (2002). Unconscious masked priming depends on temporal attention. *Psychol. Sci.* 13: 416–424.

16. Tallon-Baudry, C. (2011). On the neural mechanisms subserving consciousness and attention. *Front. Psychol.* 2: 397.

17. Baron-Cohen, S. (1995). *Mindblindness: An Essay on Autism and Theory of Mind*. Cambridge, MA: MIT Press.

18. Hoffman, E.A., and Haxby, J.V. (2000). Distinct representations of eye gaze and identity in the distributed human neural system for face perception. *Nat. Neurosci.* 3: 80–84.

19. Perrett, D.I., Smith, P.A., Potter, D.D., Mistlin, A.J., Head, A.S., Milner, A.D., and Jeeves, M.A. (1985). Visual cells in the temporal cortex sensitive to face view and gaze direction. *Proc. R. Soc. Lond. B Biol. Sci.* 223: 293–317.

20. Puce, A., Allison, T., Bentin, S., Gore, J.C., and McCarthy, G. (1998). Temporal cortex activation in humans viewing eye and mouth movements. *J. Neurosci.* 18: 2188–2199.

21. Wicker, B., Michel, F., Henaff, M.A., and Decety, J. (1998). Brain regions involved in the perception of gaze: a PET study. *Neuroimage* 8: 221–227.

22. Calder, A.J., Lawrence, A.D., Keane, J., Scott, S.K., Owen, A.M., Christoffels, I., and Young, A.W. (2002). Reading the mind from eye gaze. *Neuropsychologia* 40: 1129–1138.

23. Friesen, C.K., and Kingstone, A. (1998). The eyes have it! Reflexive orienting is triggered by nonpredictive gaze. *Psychon. Bull Rev.* 5: 490–495.

24. Kobayashi, H., and Koshima, S. (1997). Unique morphology of the human eye. *Nature* 387: 767–768.

25. Baars, B.J. (1983). Conscious contents provide the nervous system with coherent, global information. In R.J. Davidson, G.E. Schwartz, and D. Shapiro (Eds.), *Consciousness and Self Regulation*. New York: Plenum Press, p. 41.

26. Newman, J., and Baars, B.J. (1993). A neural attentional model for access to consciousness: a global workspace perspective. *Concepts Neurosci.* 4: 255–290.

27. Hofstadter, D.R. (1979). *Godel, Escher, Bach: An Eternal Golden Braid*. New York: Basic Books.

28. Haidt, J. (2005). *The Happiness Hypothesis: Finding Modern Truth in Ancient Wisdom*. New York: Basic Books.

Chapter 3: Awareness as Information

1. Descartes, R. (1641). Meditations on first philosophy. In *The Philosophical Writings of René Descartes*. Translated by J. Cottingham, R. Stoothoff, and D. Murdoch. Cambridge, UK: Cambridge University Press.

2. Kant, E. (1781). *Critique of Pure Reason*. Translated by J. M. D. Meiklejohn. Project Gutenberg. Retrieved January 22, 2013, from http://www.gutenberg.org/ebooks/4280.

3. Chalmers, D. (1995). Facing up to the problem of consciousness. *J. Conscious. Stud.* 2: 200–219.

4. Gold, J.I., and Shadlen, M.N. (2007). The neural basis of decision making. *Annu. Rev. Neurosci.* 30: 535–574.

5. Sugrue, L.P., Corrado, G.S., and Newsome, W.T. (2005). Choosing the greater of two goods: neural currencies for valuation and decision making. *Nat. Rev. Neurosci.* 6: 363–375.

6. Salzman, C.D., Britten, K.H., and Newsome, W.T. (1990). Cortical microstimulation influences perceptual judgements of motion direction. *Nature* 346: 174–177.

7. de Lafuente, V., and Ranulfo Romo, R. (2005). Neuronal correlates of subjective sensory experience. *Nat. Neurosci.* 8: 1698–1703.

8. Hernandez, A., Nacher, V., Luna, R., Zainos, A., Lemus, L., Alvarez, M., Vazquez, Y., Camarillo, L., and Romo, R. (2010). Decoding a perceptual decision process across cortex. *Neuron* 66: 300–314.

9. Newton, I. (1671). A Letter of Mr. Isaac Newton, Professor of the Mathematicks in the University of Cambridge; Containing His New Theory about Light and Colors: Sent by the Author to the Publisher from Cambridge, Febr. 6. 1671/72; In Order to be Communicated to the Royal Society. *Phil. Trans. R. Soc.* 6: 3075–3087.

10. Villamil, R. (1932). *Newton: The Man.* London: Gordon D. Knox.

11. Koch, C., and Tsuchiya, N. (2007). Attention and consciousness: two distinct brain processes. *Trends Cogn. Sci.* 11: 16–22.

12. Lamme, V.A. (2004). Separate neural definitions of visual consciousness and visual attention: a case for phenomenal awareness. *Neural Netw.* 17: 861–872.

13. O'Regan, J.K., and Noë, A. (2001). A sensorimotor account of vision and visual consciousness. *Behav. Brain Sci.* 24: 939–973.

14. Posner, M.I. (1994). Attention: the mechanisms of consciousness. *Proc. Natl. Acad. Sci. U. S. A.* 91: 7398–7403.

15. Kentridge, R.W., Heywood, C.A., and Weiskrantz, L. (2004). Spatial attention speeds discrimination without awareness in blindsight. *Neuropsychologia* 42: 831–835.

16. Naccache, L., Blandin, E., and Dehaene, S. (2002). Unconscious masked priming depends on temporal attention. *Psychol. Sci.* 13: 416–424.

17. Rock, I., Linnett, C.M., Grant, P., and Mack, A. (1992). Perception without attention: results of a new method. *Cogn. Psychol.* 24: 502–534.

Chapter 4: Being Aware Versus Knowing that You Are Aware

1. Carruthers, P. (2009). How we know our own minds: the relationship between mindreading and metacognition. *Behav. Brain Sci.* 32: 121–182.

2. Pasquali, A., Timmermans, B., Cleeremans, A. (2010). Know thyself: metacognitive networks and measures of consciousness. *Cognition* 117: 182–190.

3. Rosenthal, D.M. (2000). Consciousness, content, and metacognitive judgments. *Conscious. Cogn.* 9: 203–214.

4. Block, N. (1996). How can we find the neural correlates of consciousness? *Trends Neurosci.* 19: 456–459.

5. Dennett, D. (1991). *Consciousness Explained.* London: Penguin Press.

6. Searle, J.R. (2007). Dualism revisited. *J. Physiol. (Paris)* 101: 169–178.

7. Torczyner, H. (1979). *Magritte: Ideas and Images.* New York: New American Library.

Chapter 5: The Attention Schema

1. Johnson-Laird, P. (1983). *Mental Models.* Cambridge, UK: Cambridge University Press.

2. Beck, D.M., and Kastner, S. (2009). Top-down and bottom-up mechanisms in biasing competition in the human brain. *Vision Res.* 49: 1154–1165.

3. Desimone, R., and Duncan, J. (1995). Neural mechanisms of selective visual attention. *Annu. Rev. Neurosci.* 18: 193–222.

4. Moore, T., Armstrong, K., and Fallah, M. (2003). Visuomotor origins of covert spatial attention. *Neuron* 40: 671–683.

5. Head, H., and Holmes, G. (1911). Sensory disturbances from cerebral lesions. *Brain* 34: 102–254.

6. Graziano, M.S.A., and Botvinick, M.M. (2002). How the brain represents the body: insights from neurophysiology and psychology. In W. Prinz and B. Hommel (Eds.), *Common Mechanisms in Perception and Action: Attention and Performance XIX.* Oxford, UK: Oxford University Press, pp. 136–157.

7. Lackner, J.R. (1988). Some proprioceptive influences on the perceptual representation of body shape and orientation. *Brain* 111: 281–297.

8. Botvinick, M., and Cohen, J. (1998). Rubber hands 'feel' touch that eyes see. *Nature* 391: 756.

9. Graziano, M.S.A. (1999). Where is my arm? The relative role of vision and proprioception in the neuronal representation of limb position. *Proc. Natl. Acad. Sci. U. S. A.* 96: 10418–10421.

10. Graziano, M.S.A., Cooke, D.F., and Taylor, C.S.R. (2000). Coding the location of the arm by sight. *Science* 290: 1782–1786.

11. Petkova, V.I., and Ehrsson, H.H. (2008). If I were you: perceptual illusion of body swapping. *PLoS One* 3: e3832.

12. Hwang, E.J., Shadmehr, R. (2005). Internal models of limb dynamics and the encoding of limb state. *J. Neural Eng.* 2: S266–278.

13. Wolpert, D.M., Ghahramani, Z., and Jordan, M.I. (1995). An internal model for sensorimotor integration. *Science* 269: 1880–1882.

14. Parsons, L.M. (1987). Imagined spatial transformations of one's hands and feet. *Cogn. Psychol.* 19: 178–241.

15. Sekiyama, K. (1982). Kinesthetic aspects of mental representations in the identification of left and right hands. *Percept. Psychophys.* 32: 89–95.

16. Bonda, E., Petrides, M., Frey, S., and Evans, A. (1995). Neural correlates of mental transformations of the body-in-space. *Proc. Natl. Acad. Sci. U. S. A.* 92: 11180–11184.

17. Holland, O., and Goodman, R. (2003). Robots with internal models: a route to machine consciousness? In O. Holland (Ed.), *Machine Consciousness.* Exeter, UK: Imprint Academic, pp. 77–109.

18. Taylor, J. (2003). Paying attention to consciousness. *Prog. Neurobiol.* 71: 305–335.

Chapter 6: Illusions and Myths

1. Irwin, H.J. (1985). *Flight of Mind: A Psychological Study of the Out-of-Body Experience.* Lanham, MD: Scarecrow Press.

2. Ehrsson, H.H. (2007). The experimental induction of out-of-body experiences. *Science* 317: 1048.

3. Lenggenhager, B., Tadi, T., Metzinger, T., and Blanke, O. (2007). Video ergo sum: manipulating bodily self-consciousness. *Science* 317: 1096–1099.

4. Blanke, O., Ortigue, S., Landis, T., and Seeck, M. (2002). Stimulating illusory own-body perceptions. *Nature* 419: 269–270.

5. Blanke, O., and Metzinger, T. (2009). Full-body illusions and minimal phenomenal selfhood. *Trends Cogn. Sci.* 13: 7–13.

6. Coover, J.E. (1913). The feeling of being stared at. *Am. J. Psychol.* 24: 570–575.

7. Titchner, E.B. (1898). The feeling of being stared at. *Science* 8: 895–897.

8. Gross, C.G. (1999). *Brain, Vision, Memory: Tales in the History of Neuroscience.* Cambridge, MA: Bradford Books, MIT Press.

9. Dundes, A. (1981). *The Evil Eye: A Folklore Casebook.* New York: Garland Press.

10. Piaget, J. (1979). *The Child's Conception of the World.* Translated by J. Tomlinson and A. Tomlinson. Totowa, NJ: Little, Adams.

11. Cottrell, J.E., and Winer, G.A. (1994). Development in the understanding of perception: the decline of extromission perception beliefs. *Dev. Psychol.* 30: 218–228.

12. Winer, G.A., and Cottrell, J.E. (1996). Effects of drawing on directional representations of the process of vision. *J. Ed. Psychol.* 4: 704–714.

13. Winer, G.A., Cottrell, J.E., and Karefilaki, K.D. (1996). Images, words and questions: variables that influence beliefs about vision in children and adults. *J. Exp. Child Psychol.* 63: 499–525.

14. Mesmer, F.A. (1779). *Mesmerism: The Discovery of Animal Magnetism.* Translated by J. Bouler and republished in 1997. Sequim, WA: Holmes Publication Group.

15. Piccolino, M. (2006). Luigi Galvani's oath to animal electricity. *C. R. Biol.* 329: 303–318.

16. Shelley, M. (1818). *Frankenstein.* London: Lackington, Hughes, Harding, Mavor and Jones.

17. Alvarado, C.S. (2009). Late 19th- and early 20th-century discussions of animal magnetism. *Int. J. Clin. Exp. Hypn.* 57: 366–381.

18. Crabtree, A. (1993). *From Mesmer to Freud: Magnetic Sleep and the Roots of Psychological Healing.* New Haven, CT: Yale University Press

19. Benassi, V.A., Sweeney, P.D., and Drevno, G.E. (1979). Mind over matter: perceived success at psychokinesis. *J. Pers. Soc. Psychol.* 37: 1377–1386.

20. Langer, E.J. (1975). The illusion of control. *J. Pers. Soc. Psychol.* 32: 311–328.

21. Spence, C., Pavani, F., and Driver, J. (2000). Crossmodal links between vision and touch in covert endogenous spatial attention. *J. Exp. Psychol. Hum. Percept. Perform.* 26: 1298–2319.

Chapter 7: Social Attention

1. Baron-Cohen, S. (1995). *Mindblindness: An Essay on Autism and Theory of Mind.* Cambridge, MA: MIT Press.

2. Hoffman, E.A., and Haxby, J.V. (2000). Distinct representations of eye gaze and identity in the distributed human neural system for face perception. *Nat. Neurosci.* 3: 80–84.

3. Perrett, D.I., Smith, P.A., Potter, D.D., Mistlin, A.J., Head, A.S., Milner, A.D., and Jeeves, M.A. (1985). Visual cells in the temporal cortex sensitive to face view and gaze direction. *Proc. R. Soc. Lond. B Biol. Sci.* 223: 293–317.

4. Puce, A., Allison, T., Bentin, S., Gore, J.C., and McCarthy, G. (1998). Temporal cortex activation in humans viewing eye and mouth movements. *J. Neurosci.* 18: 2188–2199.

5. Wicker, B., Michel, F., Henaff, M.A., and Decety, J. (1998). Brain regions involved in the perception of gaze: a PET study. *Neuroimage* 8: 221–227.

6. Premack, D., and Woodruff, G. (1978). Does the chimpanzee have a theory of mind? *Behav. Brain Sci.* 1: 515–526.

7. Kobayashi, H., and Koshima, S. (1997). Unique morphology of the human eye. *Nature* 387: 767–768.

8. Yarbus, A.L. (1967). *Eye Movements and Vision.* New York: Plenum.

9. Symons, L.A., Lee, K., Cedrone, C.C., and Nishimura, M. (2004). What are you looking at? Acuity for triadic eye gaze. *J. Gen. Psychol.* 131: 451–469.

10. Calder, A.J., Lawrence, A.D., Keane, J., Scott, S.K., Owen, A.M., Christoffels, I., and Young, A.W. (2002). Reading the mind from eye gaze. *Neuropsychologia* 40: 1129–1138.

11. Posner, M.I. (1980). Orienting of attention. *Q. J. Exp. Psychol.* 32: 3–25.

12. Friesen, C.K., and Kingstone, A. (1998). The eyes have it! Reflexive orienting is triggered by nonpredictive gaze. *Psychon. Bull. Rev.* 5: 490–495.

13. Eimer, M. (1997). Uninformative symbolic cues may bias visual-spatial attention: behavioral and electrophysiological evidence. *Biol. Psychol.* 46: 67–71.

14. Ristic, J., Friesen, C.K., and Kinsgtone, A. (2002). Are eyes special? It depends on how you look at it. *Psychon. Bull. Rev.* 9: 507–513.

15. Tipples, J. (2002). Eye gaze is not unique: automatic orienting in response to uninformative arrows. *Psychon. Bull. Rev.* 9: 314–318.

16. Frischen, A., Bayliss, A.P., and Tipper, S.P. (2007). Gaze cueing of attention: visual attention, social cognition, and individual differences. *Psychol. Bull.* 133: 694–724.

Chapter 8: How Do I Distinguish My Awareness from Yours?

1. Spence, C., Pavani, F., and Driver, J. (2000). Crossmodal links between vision and touch in covert endogenous spatial attention. *J. Exp. Psychol. Hum. Percept. Perform.* 26: 1298–2319.

2. Kihlstrom, J.F. (2005). Dissociative disorders. *Annu. Rev. Clin. Psychol.* 1: 227–253.

Chapter 9: Some Useful Complexities

1. Raichle, M.E., MacLeod, A.M., Snyder, A.Z., Powers, W.J., Gusnard, D.A., Shulman, G.L. (2001). A default mode of brain function. *Proc. Natl. Acad. Sci. U. S. A.* 98: 676–682.

2. Raichle, M.E., Snyder, A.Z. (2007). A default mode of brain function: a brief history of an evolving idea. *Neuroimage* 37: 1083–1090.

3. Blanke, O., Ortigue, S., Landis, T., and Seeck, M. (2002). Stimulating illusory own-body perceptions. *Nature* 419: 269–270.

4. Blanke, O., and Metzinger, T. (2009). Full-body illusions and minimal phenomenal selfhood. *Trends Cogn. Sci.* 13: 7–13.

Chapter 10: Social Theories of Consciousness

1. Blackmore, S. (2011). *Consciousness: An Introduction*. New York: Oxford University Press.

2. Gazzaniga, M.S. (1970). *The Bisected Brain*. New York: Appleton Century Crofts.

3. Nisbett, R.E., and Wilson, T.D. (1977). Telling more than we can know—verbal reports on mental processes. *Psychol. Rev.* 84: 231–259.

4. Libet, B., Gleason, C.A., Wright, E.W., and Pearl, D.K. (1983). Time of conscious intention to act in relation to onset of cerebral activity (readiness-potential). The unconscious initiation of a freely voluntary act. *Brain* 106: 623–642.

5. Haggard, P. (2008). Human volition: towards a neuroscience of will. *Nat. Rev. Neurosci.* 9: 934–946.

6. Frith, C. (2002) Attention to action and awareness of other minds. *Conscious. Cogn.* 11: 481–487.

7. Ochsner, K.N., Knierim, K., Ludlow, D.H., Hanelin, J., Ramachandran, T., Glover, G., and Mackey, S.C. (2004). Reflecting upon feelings: an fMRI study of neural systems supporting the attribution of emotion to self and other. *J. Cogn. Neurosci.* 16: 1746–1772.

8. Saxe, R., Moran, J.M., Scholz, J., and Gabrieli, J. (2006). Overlapping and non-overlapping brain regions for theory of mind and self reflection in individual subjects. *Soc. Cogn. Affect. Neurosci.* 1: 229–234.

9. Vogeley, K., Bussfeld, P., Newen, A., Herrmann, S., Happé, F., Falkai, P., Maier, W., Shah, N.J., Fink, G.R., and Zilles, K. (2001). Mind reading: neural mechanisms of theory of mind and self-perspective. *Neuroimage* 14: 170–181.

10. Vogeley, K., May, M., Ritzl, A., Falkai, P., Zilles, K., and Fink, G.R. (2004). Neural correlates of first-person perspective as one constituent of human self-consciousness. *J. Cogn. Neurosci.* 16: 817–827.

11. Frith, C. (1995). Consciousness is for other people. *Behav. Brain Sci.* 18: 682–683.

12. Humphrey, N. (1983). *Consciousness Regained: Chapters in the Development of Mind*. Oxford, UK: Oxford University Press.

13. Noe, A. (2009). *Out of Our Heads*. New York: Hill and Wang.

14. Kanner, L. (1943). Autistic disturbances of affective contact. *Nerv. Child* 2: 217–250.

15. Volkmar, F., Chawarska, K., and Klin, A. (2005). Autism in infancy and early childhood. *Annu. Rev. Psychol.* 56: 315–336.

16. Hill, E., Berthoz, S., and Frith, U. (2004). Cognitive processing of own emotions in individuals with autistic spectrum disorders and in their relatives. *J. Autism Dev. Disord.* 34: 229–235.

17. Curtiss, S. (1977). *Genie. A Psycholinguistic Study of a Modern Day "Wild Child"*. London: Academic Press.

18. Koluchova, J. (1972). Severe deprivation in twins: a case study. *J. Child Psychol. Psychiatry* 13: 107–114.

19. Skuse, D. (1984). Extreme deprivation in early childhood. Diverse outcomes for three siblings from an extraordinary family. *J. Child Psychol. Psychiatry* 25: 523–541.

20. Soutter, A. (1995). Case report: successful treatment of a case of extreme isolation. *Eur. Child Adolesc. Psychiatry* 4: 39–45.

21. Chalmers, D. (1995). Facing up to the problem of consciousness. *J. Conscious. Stud.* 2: 200–219.

22. Ungerleider, L.G., and Mishkin, M. (1982).Two cortical visual systems. In D.J. Ingle, M.A. Goodale, and R.J.W. Mansfield (Eds.), *Analysis of Visual Behavior*. Cambridge, MA: MIT Press.

23. Barraclough, N.E., Xiao, D., Oram, M.W., and Perrett, D.I. (2006). The sensitivity of primate STS neurons to walking sequences and to the degree of articulation in static images. *Prog. Brain Res.* 154: 135–148.

24. Bruce, C., Desimone, R., and Gross, C.G. (1981). Visual properties of neurons in a polysensory area in superior temporal sulcus of the macaque. *J. Neurophysiol.* 46: 369–384.

25. Desimone, R., Albright, T.D., Gross, C.G., and Bruce, C. (1984). Stimulus-selective properties of inferior temporal neurons in the macaque. *J. Neurosci.* 4: 2051–2062.

26. Gross, C.G., Bender, D.B., and Rocha-Miranda, C.E. (1969). Visual receptive fields of neurons in inferotemporal cortex of the monkey. *Science* 166: 1303–1306.

27. Jellema, T., and Perrett, D.I. (2003). Cells in monkey STS responsive to articulated body motions and consequent static posture: a case of implied motion? *Neuropsychologia* 41: 1728–1737.

28. Jellema, T., and Perrett, D.I. (2006). Neural representations of perceived bodily actions using a categorical frame of reference. *Neuropsychologia* 44: 1535–1546.

29. Perrett, D.I., Smith, P.A., Potter, D.D., Mistlin, A.J., Head, A.S., Milner, A.D., and Jeeves, M.A. (1985). Visual cells in the temporal cortex sensitive to face view and gaze direction. *Proc. R. Soc. Lond. B Biol. Sci.* 223: 293–317.

Chapter 11: Consciousness as Integrated Information

1. Baars, B.J. (1983). Conscious contents provide the nervous system with coherent, global information. In R.J. Davidson, G.E. Schwartz, and D. Shapiro (Eds.), *Consciousness and Self Regulation.* New York: Plenum Press, p. 41.

2. Newman, J., and Baars, B.J. (1993). A neural attentional model for access to consciousness: a global workspace perspective. *Concepts Neurosci.* 4: 255–290.

3. Engel, A.K., König, P., Gray, C.M., and Singer, W. (1990). Stimulus-dependent neuronal oscillations in cat visual cortex: inter-columnar interaction as determined by cross-correlation analysis. *Eur. J. Neurosci.* 2: 588–606.

4. Engel, A.K., and Singer, W. (2001). Temporal binding and the neural correlates of sensory awareness. *Trends Cogn. Sci.* 5: 16–25.

5. Fries, P. (2009). Neuronal gamma-band synchronization as a fundamental process in cortical computation. *Annu. Rev. Neurosci.* 32: 209–224.

6. Palva, S., and Palva, J.M. (2007). New vistas for alpha-frequency band oscillations. *Trends Neurosci.* 30: 150–158.

7. Schroeder, C.E., Wilson, D.A., Radman, T., Scharfman, H., and Lakatos, P. (2010). Dynamics of active sensing and perceptual selection. *Curr. Opin. Neurobiol.* 20: 172–176

8. Crick, F., and Koch, C. (1990). Toward a neurobiological theory of consciousness. *Semin. Neurosci.* 2: 263–275.

9. Damasio, A.R. (1990). Synchronous activation in multiple cortical regions: a mechanism for recall. *Semin. Neurosci.* 2: 287–296.

10. Grossberg, S. (1999). The link between brain learning, attention, and consciousness. *Conscious. Cogn.* 8: 1–44.

11. Lamme, V.A. (2006). Towards a true neural stance on consciousness. *Trends Cogn. Sci.* 10: 494–501.

12. Llinas, R., and Ribary, U. (1994). Perception as an oneiric-like state modulated by the senses. In C. Koch and J. Davis (Eds.), *Large Scale Neural Theories of the Brain*. Cambridge, MA: MIT Press, pp. 111–124.

13. Von der Malsburg, C. (1997). The coherence definition of consciousness. In M. Ito, Y. Miyashita, and E. Rolls (Eds.), *Cognition, Computation, and Consciousness*. New York: Oxford University Press, pp. 193–204.

14. Tononi, G. (2008). Consciousness as integrated information: a provisional manifesto. *Biol. Bull.* 215: 216–242.

15. Tononi, G., and Edelman, G.M. (1998). Consciousness and complexity. *Science* 282: 1846–1851.

16. Goodale, M.A., and Milner, A.D. (1992). Separate visual pathways for perception and action. *Trends Neurosci.* 15: 20–25

17. Westwood, D.A., and Goodale, M.A. (2010). Converging evidence for diverging pathways: neuropsychology and psychophysics tell the same story. *Vision Res.* 51: 804–811.

18. Kouider, S., and Dehaene, S. (2007). Levels of processing during non-conscious perception: a critical review of visual masking. *Phil. Trans. R. Soc. Lond. B Biol. Sci.* 362: 857–875.

19. Koch, C., and Crick, F. (2001). The zombie within. *Nature* 411: 893.

Chapter 12: Neural Correlates of Consciousness

1. Blake, R., and Logothetis, N.K. (2002). Visual competition. *Nat. Rev. Neurosci.* 3: 13–21.

2. Crick, F., and Koch, C. (1998). Consciousness and neuroscience. *Cereb. Cortex* 8: 97–107.

3. Tong, F., Meng, M., and Blake, R. (2006). Neural bases of binocular rivalry. *Trends Cogn. Sci.* 10: 502–511.

4. Leopold, D.A., and Logothetis, N.K. (1996). Activity changes in early visual cortex reflect monkeys' percepts during binocular rivalry. *Nature* 379: 549–553.

5. Schurger, A., Pereira, F., Treisman, A., and Cohen, J.D. (2010). Reproducibility distinguishes conscious from nonconscious neural representations. *Science* 327: 97–99.

6. Weiskrantz, L., Warrington, E.K., Sanders, M.D., and Marshall, J. (1974). Visual capacity in the hemianopic field following a restricted cortical ablation. *Brain* 97: 709–728.

7. Cowey, A. (2010). The blindsight saga. *Exp. Brain Res.* 200: 3–24.

Chapter 13: Awareness and the Machinery for Social Perception

1. Desimone, R., Albright, T.D., Gross, C.G., and Bruce, C. (1984). Stimulus-selective properties of inferior temporal neurons in the macaque. *J. Neurosci.* 4: 2051–2062.

2. Gross, C.G., Bender, D.B., and Rocha-Miranda, C.E. (1969). Visual receptive fields of neurons in inferotemporal cortex of the monkey. *Science* 166: 1303–1306.

3. Barraclough, N.E., Xiao, D., Oram, M.W., and Perrett, D.I. (2006). The sensitivity of primate STS neurons to walking sequences and to the degree of articulation in static images. *Prog. Brain Res.* 154: 135–148.

4. Bruce, C., Desimone, R., and Gross, C.G. (1981). Visual properties of neurons in a polysensory area in superior temporal sulcus of the macaque. *J. Neurophysiol.* 46: 369–384.

5. Jellema, T., and Perrett, D.I. (2003). Cells in monkey STS responsive to articulated body motions and consequent static posture: a case of implied motion? *Neuropsychologia* 41: 1728–1737.

6. Jellema, T., and Perrett, D.I. (2006). Neural representations of perceived bodily actions using a categorical frame of reference. *Neuropsychologia* 44: 1535–1546.

7. Perrett, D.I., Smith, P.A., Potter, D.D., Mistlin, A.J., Head, A.S., Milner, A.D., and Jeeves, M.A. (1985). Visual cells in the temporal cortex sensitive to face view and gaze direction. *Proc. R. Soc. Lond. B Biol. Sci.* 223: 293–317.

8. Kanwisher, N., McDermott, J., and Chun, M.M. (1997). The fusiform face area: a module in human extrastriate cortex specialized for face perception. *J. Neurosci.* 17: 4302–4311.

9. Grossman, E., Donnelly, M., Price, R., Pickens, D., Morgan, V., Neighbor, G., and Blake, R. (2000). Brain areas involved in perception of biological motion. *J. Cogn. Neurosci.* 12: 711–720.

10. Pelphrey, K.A., Morris, J.P., Michelich, C.R., Allison, T., and McCarthy, G. (2005). Functional anatomy of biological motion perception in posterior temporal cortex: an FMRI study of eye, mouth and hand movements. *Cereb. Cortex* 15: 1866–1876.

11. Puce, A., Allison, T., Bentin, S., Gore, J.C., and McCarthy, G. (1998). Temporal cortex activation in humans viewing eye and mouth movements. *J. Neurosci.* 18: 2188–2199.

12. Thompson, J.C., Hardee, J.E., Panayiotou, A., Crewther, D., and Puce, A. (2007). Common and distinct brain activation to viewing dynamic sequences of face and hand movements. *Neuroimage* 37: 966–973.

13. Vaina, L.M., Solomon, J., Chowdhury, S., Sinha, P., and Belliveau, J.W. (2001). Functional neuroanatomy of biological motion perception in humans. *Proc. Natl. Acad. Sci. U. S. A.* 98: 11656–11661.

14. Wicker, B., Michel, F., Henaff, M.A., and Decety, J. (1998). Brain regions involved in the perception of gaze: a PET study. *Neuroimage* 8: 221–227.

15. Wyk, B.C., Hudac, C.M., Carter, E.J., Sobel, D.M., and Pelphrey, K.A. (2009). Action understanding in the superior temporal sulcus region. *Psychol. Sci.* 20: 771–777.

16. Pelphrey, K.A., Morris, J.P., and McCarthy, G. (2004). Grasping the intentions of others: the perceived intentionality of an action influences activity in the superior temporal sulcus during social perception. *J. Cogn. Neurosci.* 16: 1706–1716.

17. Blakemore, S.J., Boyer, P., Pachot-Clouard, M., Meltzoff, A., Segebarth, C., and Decety, J. (2003). The detection of contingency and animacy from simple animations in the human brain. *Cereb. Cortex* 13: 837–844.

18. Frith, U., and Frith, C.D. (2003). Development and neurophysiology of mentalizing. *Phil. Trans. R. Soc. Lond. B Biol. Sci.* 358: 459–473.

19. Premack, D., and Woodruff, G. (1978). Does the chimpanzee have a theory of mind? *Behav. Brain Sci.* 1: 515–526.

20. Wimmer, H., and Perner, J. (1983). Beliefs about beliefs: representation and constraining function of wrong beliefs in young children's understanding of deception. *Cognition* 13: 103–128.

21. Brunet, E., Sarfati, Y., Hardy-Baylé, M.C., and Decety, J. (2000). A PET investigation of the attribution of intentions with a nonverbal task. *Neuroimage* 11: 157–166.

22. Ciaramidaro, A., Adenzato, M., Enrici, I., Erk, S., Pia, L., Bara, B.G., and Walter, H. (2007). The intentional network: how the brain reads varieties of intentions. *Neuropsychologia* 45: 3105–3113.

23. Fletcher, P.C., Happé, F., Frith, U., Baker, S.C., Dolan, R.J., Frackowiak, R.S., and Frith, C.D. (1995). Other minds in the brain: a functional imaging study of "theory of mind" in story comprehension. *Cognition* 57: 109–128.

24. Gallagher, H.L., Happé, F., Brunswick, N., Fletcher, P.C., Frith, U., and Frith, C.D. (2000). Reading the mind in cartoons and stories: an fMRI study of 'theory of mind' in verbal and nonverbal tasks. *Neuropsychologia* 38: 11–21.

25. Goel, V., Grafman, J., Sadato, N., and Hallett, M. (1995). Modeling other minds. *Neuroreport* 6: 1741–1746.

26. Saxe, R., and Kanwisher, N. (2003). People thinking about thinking people: fMRI investigations of theory of mind. *Neuroimage* 19: 1835–1842.

27. Saxe, R., and Wexler, A. (2005). Making sense of another mind: the role of the right temporo-parietal junction. *Neuropsychologia* 43: 1391–1399.

28. Vogeley, K., Bussfeld, P., Newen, A., Herrmann, S., Happé, F., Falkai, P., Maier, W., Shah, N.J., Fink, G.R., and Zilles, K. (2001). Mind reading: neural mechanisms of theory of mind and self-perspective. *Neuroimage* 14: 170–181.

29. Astafiev, S.V., Shulman, G.L., and Corbetta, M. (2006). Visuospatial reorienting signals in the human temporo-parietal junction are independent of response selection. *Eur. J. Neurosci.* 23: 591–596.

30. Corbetta, M., Kincade, J.M., Ollinger, J.M., McAvoy, M.P., and Shulman, G.L. (2000). Voluntary orienting is dissociated from target detection in human posterior parietal cortex. *Nat. Neurosci.* 3: 292–297.

31. Shulman, G.L., Pope, D.L., Astafiev, S.V., McAvoy, M.P., Snyder, A.Z., and Corbetta, M. (2010). Right hemisphere dominance during spatial selective attention and target detection occurs outside the dorsal frontoparietal network. *J. Neurosci.* 30: 3640–3651.

32. Mitchell, L.P. (2008). Activity in the right temporo-parietal junction is not selective for theory-of-mind. *Cereb. Cortex* 18: 262–271.

33. Rizzolatti, G., and Sinigaglia, C. (2010). The functional role of the parieto-frontal mirror circuit: interpretations and misinterpretations. *Nat. Rev. Neurosci.* 11: 264–274.

34. Descartes, R. (1641). Meditations on first philosophy. In *The Philosophical Writings of René Descartes*. Translated by J. Cottingham, R. Stoothoff, and D. Murdoch. Cambridge, UK: Cambridge University Press.

35. Passingham, R.E., Bengtsson, S.L., and Lau, H.C. (2010). Medial frontal cortex: from self-generated action to reflection on one's own performance. *Trends Cogn. Sci.* 14: 16–21.

36. Frith, C. (2002) Attention to action and awareness of other minds. *Conscious. Cogn.* 11: 481–487.

37. Ochsner, K.N., Knierim, K., Ludlow, D.H., Hanelin, J., Ramachandran, T., Glover, G., and Mackey, S.C. (2004). Reflecting upon feelings: an fMRI study of neural systems supporting the attribution of emotion to self and other. *J. Cog. Neurosci.* 16: 1746–1772.

38. Saxe, R., Moran, J.M., Scholz, J., and Gabrieli, J. (2006). Overlapping and non-overlapping brain regions for theory of mind and self reflection in individual subjects. *Soc. Cogn. Affect. Neurosci.* 1: 229–234.

39. Vogeley, K., May, M., Ritzl, A., Falkai, P., Zilles, K., and Fink, G.R. (2004). Neural correlates of first-person perspective as one constituent of human self-consciousness. *J. Cogn. Neurosci.* 16: 817–827.

40. Raichle, M.E., MacLeod, A.M., Snyder, A.Z., Powers, W.J., Gusnard, D.A., Shulman, G.L. (2001). A default mode of brain function. *Proc. Natl. Acad. Sci. U. S. A.* 98: 676–682.

41. Raichle, M.E., Snyder, A.Z. (2007). A default mode of brain function: a brief history of an evolving idea. *Neuroimage* 37: 1083–1090.

42. Karnath, H.O., Ferber, S., and Himmelbach, M. (2001). Spatial awareness is a function of the temporal not the posterior parietal lobe. *Nature* 411: 950–953.

43. Vallar, G., and Perani, D. (1986). The anatomy of unilateral neglect after right-hemisphere stroke lesions. A clinical/CT-scan correlation study in man. *Neuropsychologia* 24: 609–622.

Chapter 14: The Neglect Syndrome

1. Brain, W.R. (1941). A form of visual disorientation resulting from lesions of the right cerebral hemisphere. *Proc. R. Soc. Med.* 34: 771–776.

2. Critchley, M. (1953). *The Parietal Lobes.* London: Hafner Press.

3. Bisiach, E., and Luzzatti, C. (1978). Unilateral neglect of representational space. *Cortex* 14: 129–133.

4. Berti, A., and Rizzolatti, G. (1992). Visual processing without awareness: evidence from unilateral neglect. *J. Cogn. Neurosci.* 4: 345–351.

5. McGlinchey-Berroth, R., Milberg, W.P., Verfaellie, M., Alexander, M., and Kilduff, P. (1993). Semantic priming in the neglected field: evidence from a lexical decision task. *Cogn. Neuropsychol.* 10: 79–108.

6. Marshall, J.C., and Halligan, P.W. (1988). Blindsight and insight in visuo-spatial neglect. *Nature* 336: 766–767.

7. Rees, G., Wojciulik, E., Clarke, K., Husain, M., Frith, C., and Driver, J. (2000). Unconscious activation of visual cortex in the damaged right hemisphere of a parietal patient with extinction. *Brain* 123: 1624–1633.

8. Vuilleumier, P., Armony, J.L., Clarke K., Husain, M., Driver, J., Dolan, R.J. (2002). Neural response to emotional faces with and without awareness: event-related fMRI in a parietal patient with visual extinction and spatial neglect. *Neuropsychologia* 40: 2156–2166.

9. Mort, D.J., Malhotra, P., Mannan, S.K., Rorden, C., Pambakian, A., Kennard, C., and Husain, M. (2003). The anatomy of visual neglect. *Brain* 126: 1986–1997.

10. Beck, D.M., and Kastner, S. (2009). Top-down and bottom-up mechanisms in biasing competition in the human brain. *Vision Res.* 49: 1154–1165.

11. Heilman, K.M., and Valenstein, E. (1972). Frontal lobe neglect in man. *Neurology* 22: 660–664.

12. Mesulam, M.M. (1999). Spatial attention and neglect: parietal, frontal and cingulate contributions to the mental representation and attentional targeting of salient extrapersonal events. *Phil. Trans. R. Soc. Lond. B Biol. Sci.* 354: 1325–1346.

13. Ptak, R., and Schnider, A. (2010). The dorsal attention network mediates orienting toward behaviorally relevant stimuli in spatial neglect. *J. Neurosci.* 30: 12557–12565.

14. Vallar, G., and Perani, D. (1986). The anatomy of unilateral neglect after right-hemisphere stroke lesions. A clinical/CT-scan correlation study in man. *Neuropsychologia* 24: 609–622.

15. Ferber, S., and Karnath, H.O. (2001). How to assess spatial neglect-line bisection or cancellation tasks. *J. Clin. Exp. Neuropsychol.* 23: 599–607.

16. Karnath, H.O., Ferber, S., and Himmelbach, M. (2001). Spatial awareness is a function of the temporal not the posterior parietal lobe. *Nature* 411: 950–953.

17. Rorden, C., Fruhmann Berger, M., and Karnath, H.O. (2006). Disturbed line bisection is associated with posterior brain lesions. *Brain Res.* 1080: 17–25.

18. Halligan, P.W., and Marshall, J.C. (1992). Left visuo-spatial neglect: a meaningless entity? *Cortex* 28: 525–535.

19. Halligan, P.W., Fink, G.R., Marshall, J.C., and Vallar, G. (2003). Spatial cognition: evidence from visual neglect. *Trends Cogn. Sci.* 7: 125–133.

20. Vallar, G. (2001). Extrapersonal visual unilateral spatial neglect and its neuroanatomy. *Neuroimage* 14: S52–S58.

21. Carruthers, P. (2011). Should damage to the social machinery damage perception? *Cogn. Neurosci.* 2: 116–117.

22. Apperly, I.A., Samson, D., Chiavarino, C., and Humphreys, G.W. (2004). Frontal and temporo-parietal lobe contributions to theory of mind: neuropsychological evidence from a false-belief task with reduced language and executive demands. *J. Cogn. Neurosci.* 16: 1773–1784.

23. Samson, D., Apperly, I.A., Chiavarino, C., and Humphreys, G.W. (2004). Left temporoparietal junction is necessary for representing someone else's belief. *Nat. Neurosci.* 7: 499–500.

24. Weed, E., McGregor, W., Feldbaek Nielsen, J., Roepstorff, A., and Frith, U. (2010). Theory of mind in adults with right hemisphere damage: what's the story? *Brain Lang.* 113: 65–72.

25. Heilman, K.M., and Valenstein, E. (1972). Mechansism underlying hemispatial neglect. *Ann. Neurol.* 5: 166–170.

26. Mesulam, M.M. (1981). A cortical network for directed attention and unilateral neglect. *Ann. Neurol.* 10: 309–325.

27. Kinsbourne, M. (1970). A model for the mechanism of unilateral neglect of space. *Trans. Am. Neurol. Assoc.* 95: 143–146.

28. Szczepanski, S.M., Konen, C.S., and Kastner, S. (2010). Mechanisms of spatial attention control in frontal and parietal cortex. *J. Neurosci.* 30: 148–160.

Chapter 15: Multiple Interlocking Functions of the Brain Area TPJ

1. Astafiev, S.V., Shulman, G.L., and Corbetta, M. (2006). Visuospatial reorienting signals in the human temporo-parietal junction are independent of response selection. *Eur. J. Neurosci.* 23: 591–596.

2. Corbetta, M., Kincade, J.M., Ollinger, J.M., McAvoy, M.P., and Shulman, G.L. (2000). Voluntary orienting is dissociated from target detection in human posterior parietal cortex. *Nat. Neurosci.* 3: 292–297.

3. Shulman, G.L., Pope, D.L., Astafiev, S.V., McAvoy, M.P., Snyder, A.Z., and Corbetta, M. (2010). Right hemisphere dominance during spatial selective attention and target detection occurs outside the dorsal frontoparietal network. *J. Neurosci.* 30: 3640–3651.

4. Scholz, J., Triantafyllou, C., Whitfield-Gabrieli, S., Brown, E.N., and Saxe, R. (2009). Distinct regions of right temporo-parietal junction are selective for theory of mind and exogenous attention. *PLoS One* 4: e4869.

5. Aflalo, T.N., and Graziano, M.S.A. (2011). The organization of the macaque extrastriate visual cortex re-examined using the principle of spatial continuity of function. *J. Neurophysiol.* 105: 305–320.

6. Graziano, M.S.A., and Aflalo, T.N. (2007). Rethinking cortical organization: moving away from discrete areas arranged in hierarchies. *Neuroscientist* 13: 138–147.

7. Addis, D.R., Wong, A.T., and Schacter, D.L. (2007). Remembering the past and imagining the future: common and distinct neural substrates during event construction and elaboration. *Neuropsychologia* 45: 1363–1377.

8. Hassabis, D., Kumaran, D., and Maguire, E.A. (2007). Using imagination to understand the neural basis of episodic memory. *J. Neurosci.* 27: 14365–14374.

9. Rabin, J.S., Gilboa, A., Stuss, D.T., Mar, R.A., Rosenbaum, R.S. (2010). Common and unique neural correlates of autobiographical memory and theory of mind. *J. Cogn. Neurosci.* 22: 1095–1111.

10. Blanke, O., Ortigue, S., Landis, T., and Seeck, M. (2002). Stimulating illusory own-body perceptions. *Nature* 419: 269–270.

11. Fletcher, P.C., Happé, F., Frith, U., Baker, S.C., Dolan, R.J., Frackowiak, R.S., and Frith, C.D. (1995). Other minds in the brain: a functional imaging study of "theory of mind" in story comprehension. *Cognition* 57: 109–128.

12. Gallagher, H.L., Happé, F., Brunswick, N., Fletcher, P.C., Frith, U., and Frith, C.D. (2000). Reading the mind in cartoons and stories: an fMRI study of 'theory of mind' in verbal and nonverbal tasks. *Neuropsychologia* 38: 11–21.

13. Goel, V., Grafman, J., Sadato, N., and Hallett, M. (1995). Modeling other minds. *Neuroreport* 6: 1741–1746.

14. Saxe, R., and Kanwisher, N. (2003). People thinking about thinking people: fMRI investigations of theory of mind. *Neuroimage* 19: 1835–1842.

15. Saxe, R., and Wexler, A. (2005). Making sense of another mind: the role of the right temporo-parietal junction. *Neuropsychologia* 43: 1391–1399.

16. Vogeley, K., Bussfeld, P., Newen, A., Herrmann, S., Happé, F., Falkai, P., Maier, W., Shah, N.J., Fink, G.R., and Zilles, K. (2001). Mind reading: neural mechanisms of theory of mind and self-perspective. *Neuroimage* 14: 170–181.

17. Grossman, E., Donnelly, M., Price, R., Pickens, D., Morgan, V., Neighbor, G., and Blake, R. (2000). Brain areas involved in perception of biological motion. *J. Cogn. Neurosci.* 12: 711–720.

18. Pelphrey, K.A., Morris, J.P., Michelich, C.R., Allison, T., and McCarthy, G. (2005). Functional anatomy of biological motion perception in posterior temporal cortex: an FMRI study of eye, mouth and hand movements. *Cereb. Cortex* 15: 1866–1876.

19. Puce, A., Allison, T., Bentin, S., Gore, J.C., and McCarthy, G. (1998). Temporal cortex activation in humans viewing eye and mouth movements. *J. Neurosci.* 18: 2188–2199.

20. Thompson, J.C., Hardee, J.E., Panayiotou, A., Crewther, D., and Puce, A. (2007). Common and distinct brain activation to viewing dynamic sequences of face and hand movements. *Neuroimage* 37: 966–973.

21. Vaina, L.M., Solomon, J., Chowdhury, S., Sinha, P., and Belliveau, J.W. (2001). Functional neuroanatomy of biological motion perception in humans. *Proc. Natl. Acad. Sci. U. S. A.* 98: 11656–11661.

22. Wicker, B., Michel, F., Henaff, M.A., and Decety, J. (1998). Brain regions involved in the perception of gaze: a PET study. *Neuroimage* 8: 221–227.

23. Wyk, B.C., Hudac, C.M., Carter, E.J., Sobel, D.M., and Pelphrey, K.A. (2009). Action understanding in the superior temporal sulcus region. *Psychol. Sci.* 20: 771–777.

24. Karnath, H.O., Ferber, S., and Himmelbach, M. (2001). Spatial awareness is a function of the temporal not the posterior parietal lobe. *Nature* 411: 950–953.

25. Vallar, G., and Perani, D. (1986). The anatomy of unilateral neglect after right-hemisphere stroke lesions. A clinical/CT-scan correlation study in man. *Neuropsychologia* 24: 609–622.

Chapter 16: Simulating Other Minds

1. di Pellegrino, G., Fadiga, L., Fogassi, L., Gallese, V., and Rizzolatti, G. (1992). Understanding motor events: a neurophysiological study. *Exp. Brain Res.* 91: 176–180.

2. Gallese, V., Fadiga, L., Fogassi, L., and Rizzolatti, G. (1996). Action recognition in the premotor cortex. *Brain* 119: 593–609.

3. Rizzolatti, G., Fadiga, L., Gallese, V., and Fogassi, L. (1996). Premotor cortex and the recognition of motor actions. *Brain Res. Cogn. Brain. Res.* 3: 131–141.

4. Buccino, G., Binkofski, F., Fink, G.R., Fadiga, L., Fogassi, L., Gallese, V., Seitz, R.J., Zilles, K., Rizzolatti, G., and Freund, H.J. (2001). Action observation activates premotor and parietal areas in a somatotopic manner: an fMRI study. *Eur. J. Neurosci.* 13: 400–404.

5. Filimon, F., Nelson, J.D., Hagler, D.J., and Sereno, M.I. (2007). Human cortical representations for reaching: mirror neurons for execution, observation, and imagery. *Neuroimage* 37: 1315–1328.

6. Iacoboni, M., Molnar-Szakacs, I., Gallese, V., Buccino, G., Mazziotta, J.C., and Rizzolatti, G. (2005). Grasping the intentions of others with one's own mirror neuron system. *PLoS Biol.* 3: e79.

7. Rizzolatti, G., and Sinigaglia, C. (2010). The functional role of the parieto-frontal mirror circuit: interpretations and misinterpretations. *Nat. Rev. Neurosci.* 11: 264–274.

8. Liberman, A.M., Cooper, F.S., Shankweiler, D.P., and Studdert-Kennedy, M. (1967). Perception of the speech code. *Psychol. Rev.* 74: 431–461.

9. Heyes, C. (2010). Where do mirror neurons come from? *Neurosci. Biobehav. Rev.* 34: 575–583.

10. Kilner, J.M., Friston, K.J., and Frith, C.D. (2007). Predictive coding: an account of the mirror neuron system. *Cogn. Process.* 8: 159–566.

11. Blanke, O., Ortigue, S., Landis, T., and Seeck, M. (2002). Stimulating illusory own-body perceptions. *Nature* 419: 269–270.

Chapter 17: Some Spiritual Matters

1. Dennett, D. (2006). *Breaking the Spell*. New York: Penguin Press.

2. Boyer, P. (2001). *Religion Explained: The Evolutionary Origins of Religious Thought*. New York: Basic Books.

3. Barrett, J.L. (2004). *Why Would Anyone Believe in God?* Walnut Creek, CA: AltaMira Press.

4. Atran, S. (2002). *In Gods We Trust: The Evolutionary Landscape of Religion*. New York: Oxford University Press.

5. Sosis, R., and Alcorta, C. (2003). Signaling, solidarity, and the sacred: the evolution of religious behavior. *Evolutionary Anthropology* 12: 264–274.

6. Gazzaniga, M.S. (1970). *The Bisected Brain*. New York: Appleton Century Crofts.

7. Nisbett, R.E., and Wilson, T.D. (1977). Telling more than we can know—verbal reports on mental processes. *Psychol. Rev.* 84: 231–259.

8. Libet, B., Gleason, C.A., Wright, E.W., and Pearl, D.K. (1983). Time of conscious intention to act in relation to onset of cerebral activity (readiness-potential). The unconscious initiation of a freely voluntary act. *Brain* 106: 623–642.

9. Fuhrman, M. (2005). *Silent Witness: The Untold Story of Terri Schiavo's Death*. New York: William Morrow.

10. Purves lab. Retreived January 22, 2013, from http://www.purveslab.net/seeforyourself/.

11. Purves, D. (2003). *Why We See What We Do Redux*. Sunderland, MA: Sinauer Associates.

12. Darwin, C. (1859). *On The Origin of Species by Means of Natural Selection*. London: John Murray Press.

13. Gould, S.J. (1991). Exaptation: a crucial tool for evolutionary psychology. *J. Soc. Issues* 47: 43–65.

14. Gould, S.J., and Vrba, E.S. (1982). Exaptation—a missing term in the science of form. *Paleobiology* 8: 4–15.

15. Gould, S.J., and Lewontin, R.C. (1979). The spandrels of San Marco and the Panglossian paradigm: a critique of the adaptationist programme. *Proc. R. Soc. Lond. B* 205: 581–598.

16. Frith, C. (1995). Consciousness is for other people. *Behav. Brain Sci.* 18: 682–683.

17. Humphrey, N. (1983). *Consciousness Regained: Chapters in the Development of Mind.* Oxford, UK: Oxford University Press.

18. Noe, A. (2009). *Out of Our Heads.* New York: Hill and Wang.

19. Humphrey, N. (2011). *Soul Dust.* Princeton, NJ: Princeton University Press

20. Koenig, H.G., and Cohen, H.J. (2001). *The Link between Religion and Health: Psychoneuroimmunology and the Faith Factor.* Oxford, UK: Oxford University Press.

21. Holt-Lunstad, J., Smith, T.B., Layton, J.B. (2010). Social relationships and mortality risk: a meta-analytic review. *PLoS Med.* 7: e1000316.

22. Call, J., and Tomasello, M. (2008). Does the chimpanzee have a theory of mind? 30 years later. *Trends Cogn. Sci.* 12: 187–192.

23. Hare, B., Call, J., and Tomasello, M. (2001). Do chimpanzees know what conspecifics know and do not know? *Anim. Behav.* 61: 139–151.

24. Horowitz, A. (2009). Attention to attention in domestic dog (*Canis familiaris*) dyadic play. *Anim. Cogn.* 12: 107–118.

25. Povinelli, D.J., Nelson, K.E., and Boysen, S.T. (1990). Inferences about guessing and knowing by chimpanzees (*Pan troglodytes*). *J. Comp. Psychol.* 104: 203–210.

26. Premack, D., and Woodruff, G. (1978). Does the chimpanzee have a theory of mind? *Behav. Brain Sci.* 1: 515–526.

27. Turing, A.M. (1950). Computing machinery and intelligence. *Mind* 59: 433–460.

28. Bostrum, N. (2003). Are you living in a computer simulation? *Philosophical Quarterly* 53: 243–255.

29. Dawkins, R. (2006). *The God Delusion.* New York: Houghton Mifflin Harcourt.

30. Hawking, S. (2010). *The Grand Design.* New York: Bantam.

Index